LOST WITHOUT YOU

LOST WITHOUT YOU
Loving and Losing Tanya

VINNIE JONES

SEVEN DIALS

First published in Great Britain in 2020 by Seven Dials
This paperback edition published in 2021 by Seven Dials
an imprint of The Orion Publishing Group Ltd
Carmelite House, 50 Victoria Embankment
London EC4Y 0DZ

An Hachette UK Company

1 3 5 7 9 10 8 6 4 2

A CIP catalogue record for this book is
available from the British Library.

ISBN (Mass Market Paperback) 978 1 8418 8419 6
ISBN (eBook) 978 1 8418 8420 2

Typeset by Input Data Services Ltd, Somerset

Printed in Great Britain by Clays Ltd. Elcograf S.p.A.

MIX
Paper from
responsible sources
FSC   FSC® C104740

www.orionbooks.co.uk

To Tanya
Our Sunshine

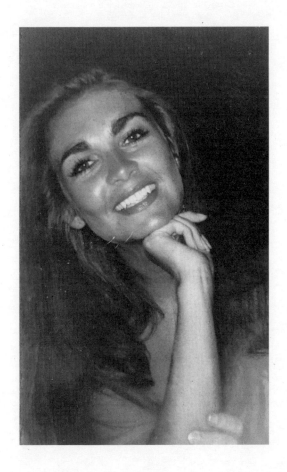

Contents

Vin has been in Los Angeles since September. I have been to visit him, but it's not the same . . . I am counting the days away. The thought of his beautiful face and his lovely smell keep me going for a while, but I miss him so much.

It's strange how you spend your whole life waiting for your special person to come along, then you find them and feel so happy, then end up living apart.

I just wish we could all just be together always.

Tanya Jones, 19 October 2000

Prologue:
WHERE DO I BEGIN?

This is not a love story I ever wanted to tell, because I hoped it would just go on and on, and never end, and never be a story – I thought it would always just *be*, and that we'd grow old together. I never wanted it to be a tale I told about the *past*, a middle-aged man sitting at the kitchen table as the California light fades, thinking about the coming night and how to get through it, and trying to explain to someone – to anyone – what it was like to live through something extraordinary, an amazing three decades that happened to me, three decades that are now over.

I don't feel this way because the *love story* is over; I'll always love Tanya Lamont, who became Tanya Jones, who was always just my beautiful Tans. No – the love I feel for her is *present*, and *real*, and will never fade. So, the feeling is there, and will always be there . . . but she is gone from this world and I'm left here. Her body finally failed her, failed all of us, and we're left with photographs and memories and sometimes we sneak into her closet to smell her clothes, the scent she wore, though it's fading, every day it's fading fast.

1

I cling on to some things; like the last card she gave to me. Inside she'd written:

To my love Vin, something wonderful happens to me every day. It's being with you. You are my morning sunshine the moment I wake. All my love, Tanya.

How do you live without that? If anyone can tell me, I'd happily listen. She wrote that card after we'd been together 27 years – and I've been hard to live with at times. But every day she still looked at me and saw something wonderful.

I sometimes tell people that I'm just waiting to be reunited with Tans. In one interview I said, 'I'm going to get on with my life, I'm going to crash through it, but in terms of the universe, it would be the smallest dot, that's how I look at it. Basically, I've got a few years to wait now until we're back together.'

I suppose in some ways I'm just hanging around, half-living, until I get to see her again. Everyone tries to talk me out of it – 'You're not old, Vin,' they say, 'You're healthy, you have lots of time left', but it's how I feel some days. I'm just waiting, kicking my heels, passing the time, keeping busy, hitting fucking golf balls into a sea of sadness. Grief is like that: a great, heavy weight, heavier than any element, so heavy it can sink through the table and the floor and through the basement of the house and down into the deep rock. And some days, it takes you with it. And it's on those days that I tell people I'm just waiting to be reunited with Tanya Jones.

I was talking to a guy at the golf course the other day and he told me that his wife had passed away 14 years earlier. We both went quiet – it's a horrible club to be part of, and no amount of 'I'm sorry's can make anyone feel better, not really. But I tried; I told him I was so sorry, just as he'd told me he was sorry when he learned about Tans.

I was just about to walk away when the guy stopped me and said, 'It doesn't get any easier, you know.'

Just like that. Nothing else, just that.

I said, 'Sorry?'

'You learn to live with it,' he said, 'but it doesn't get any easier. Sure, you learn to suspend the grief because it's so heavy. That's what you do. But no, mate. It doesn't get any easier.'

So yeah, some days the light at the end of the tunnel is that it won't be long until we're together. No, I'm not an old man, not quite, and no, that's not all I feel. There are days I look up and tell her what I'm up to, and try to make her laugh, or at least to put a smile on her face. The way I'm looking at it is this: she's up there now, sitting there, looking down on us, so I try to be a good person. I know I have a reputation for some of the things I've done, but you've no idea how much I've changed. A lot of the time I try to do something good for people, and when I do good things, I feel her smiling. I know that smile – I lived with it for 27 years.

I know that smile.

I'm writing this book because I want people to understand what grief does, and maybe how to cope with it.

I'm no expert – Tanya only died in the last year, and I'm still trying to find my way through the heavy, dark, painful rain that seems to fall every single day, even in sunny southern California. I hope I never become an expert to be honest; it's too hard. But I'm learning to deal with it the best I can.

The nights are really tough, I'll tell you that for nothing. I can keep myself busy through the days – I'm acting, and making movies, and doing deals, and appearances, and singing on *The X Factor*, and playing golf, and hanging out with Tans' daughter, Kaley, and seeing my friends and family back in the UK.

Kaley is buying a house with her partner, and that's been a great distraction. When Kaley moves into that house, I know I can look up and feel Tans' loving smile – I know how she's going to react; it was one of the things she most wanted at the end, for Kaley and her partner to be settled in their own place.

But the nights . . . that's when the loneliness hits hardest. I think of all the times we'd snuggle down to watch the telly, holding hands, going over the day, laughing at something someone said – those secret moments that make a relationship. No one can ever know what happens between two people, not really, and no one can know because no one can truly understand what happens in those private, intimate moments – two friends lying next to each other, being honest, being vulnerable, being gentle, being happy. Not having that any more . . . the pain is like a fire you don't want to touch, or even get too close to.

Twenty years ago, Tans wrote in a diary about how strange it is to spend your whole life waiting to meet someone special, and how when you do finally find them, you're happy, but then you can end up living apart. She was talking about me spending time in the States when my acting career took off but I re-read those words now and think she might have had some kind of premonition.

In fact, we both faced the prospect of being apart all through our relationship. That's because in 1987, Tanya's heart had collapsed as she gave birth to Kaley which meant she'd had to have a heart transplant, so we were never sure how long she had to live.

But her heart was fine, right up to the end. It pumped, yes, but it was also full of love and laughter and kindness.

I think about her heart every morning when I wake up. I'm up every day at half past five; boom, let's go. The first thing I do is make my bed – I get up and I make the bed – and I hadn't done that in 27 years, I'm embarrassed to admit. I decided to do that because, just after we lost Tans, I happened to watch a graduation speech given at the University of Texas by a guy called William H. McRaven, who is a retired United States Navy four-star admiral – a tough fella who oversaw the capture of Saddam Hussein, the rescue of Captain Phillips from the Somali pirates, and the killing of bin Laden. So, he's not exactly a pussy cat, this fella, but with all that experience, what was the first thing he said? You might imagine it was something about being brave or standing up for what you believe in or whatever. Well, it wasn't any of that – instead, it was, 'If you want to change

5

the world, start off by making your bed.' Because it doesn't matter how bad your day is going to be, as McRaven put it, 'If by chance you have a miserable day, you will come home to a bed that is made.' So, if it was good enough for the guy whose forces threw bin Laden into the North Arabian Sea, it was good enough for me.

As I'm doing my hospital corners, I have a little chat with Tans and make sure it's alright. That's how I start the day off: I make the bed, and I have a chat with her. Every single day. I say to her, 'Let's do this today, Tans,' or, 'I'm going to do that.' I even check with her about my bed-making skills – I'll say, 'Is the bed alright? Hold on a minute. I didn't do that bit like I should have!' and I have a bit of a giggle with her. We laugh every day. And I've gotten really good at making a bed.

I have these conversations in my mind, mostly, but some days, I say these things out loud, into the air, where she is.

And then the day is on – I crash through it, keeping busy.

Tans keeps me strong, and the memory of her love has helped me realize important things, like you've got to keep getting out there for other people who are struggling. Whenever you think you've got a problem, there's always someone around the corner in more trouble. That's why you have to talk about what's happening, and you have to turn to your friends. I've got an amazing group of pals, and they're not celebrity friends, though I have some of those too. But my dearest are the people I grew up with around Watford, Hemel Hempstead, Bedmond, places like that. I've met great friends along the way as I've travelled to play football and to act and to do my businesses, but it's that original group that I've found myself leaning on the most. They're the people you turn to; they're the ones that knew me before Tans, during Tans and will know me forever.

The hardest part to adjust to is that everybody's life goes on. When you're facing the biggest tragedy of your life, they're still going to work, coming back from work, queuing up for Starbucks. The enormity of it all is so heavy. I keep opening the paper and putting on the TV and I can't believe that she's still not the lead item on every page, on every broadcast. That disconnect between the personal tragedy and the spinning earth is a really hard one to navigate. I keep thinking of that poem that John Hannah reads in *Four Weddings and a Funeral* (Tans loved it), the one that goes, 'Stop all the clocks, cut off the telephone'.

That's exactly how it feels, when someone dies, someone you've lived with for half of your life. You can't believe time continues; you can't understand why people are just walking down the street doing their usual things. Sometimes I want to stop people as they pass and shake them awake and tell them that the worst possible thing has happened . . . and then I remember that it only feels that way to me, and Kaley, and Tans' parents and brother, and her closest friends.

So somehow you have to turn these negatives into positives so you can move forward in life and not be swallowed up by the great whale that is grief. Tans told us before she died that she'd be waiting for us and I truly believe that;

for me, that's a great positive, a thought that I cling to. The idea that I'll see her again is something so powerful that I find myself looking forward to it; not in a morbid way, but in a way that gives me a little spring in my step; just a little spring, but I'll take it. I think that's the best way to deal with it.

Tans said that the beautiful thing for her was waking up with me. I know there's times I was a bugger, but Tans felt safe with me – whatever problems came up, I could deal with them; we dealt with them together.

Until a final meeting in a room in Cedars-Sinai Medical Center where I couldn't fix the problems any longer.

I realize our time on this planet – everyone's time – is minute compared to the vast sweep of human history. We're just a blip, a tiny accident of mathematics. Some brilliant scientist said that if you calculated the chances of your ancestors meeting and having kids, and then all the way down to your parents – and don't forget they have to meet, and the right egg and the right sperm have to get together, and all that – well, the chances it'll happen, expressed as a number, is basically zero. This doctor – Dr Ali Binazir – said:

> [The chances of one person existing] is the probability of two million people getting together each to play a game of dice with trillion-sided dice. They each roll the dice and they all come up with the exact same number – for example, 550,343,279,001. A miracle is an event so unlikely as to be almost impossible. Now go forth and feel and act like the miracle that you are.

Now, add on top of that the impossibility that is one Vinnie and one Tans, and they have to meet, and lose contact, and meet again, and lose contact, and end up moving in next door to each other, and get married ... Well, I'm proud to say that we *did* live like it was a miracle.

But it wasn't because of maths; it had nothing to do with science of DNA or any of that. It was just a miracle, a throw of a big dice that came up showing a six every single minute of every single day.

Tans spent hundreds of nights in hospital beds, but she never spent one on her own. Not one. I was there every single night. She was in intensive care a lot, but she never woke up to find me gone. That's why I believe she's with me now, all the time; she will never leave my side, so I never wake up alone, either.

Except, I wake up alone every day.

Someone asked me recently who was looking after me, now that Tans is gone.

I said, 'The power of her love, that's what looks after me.'

But for all the making of the beds and crashing through the days and keeping busy, deep down this is what it feels like: I'm underwater; I can't tell if I'm a few inches below the surface, or five feet, or a thousand metres, or one hundred miles. It is not dark. There is sunlight streaming down, but I have no buoyancy and I can't get myself to the air. I reach my hand up towards the light, but it never quite reaches; I never manage to break the surface.

I feel like the bed covers are 40 feet deep on top of me ...

I guess this means I'm drowning. This is it, then. You

can't hear, you can't have conversations – sound is all numbed out, muffled.

All the struggle and fame and fights and matches and films and drinks and premieres and interviews and *Big Brother* and *X Factor* and my childhood and nights in the cells and Aaron and Kaley and my mum and dad and Tans . . . all of it, slipping away as the water surrounds me. It doesn't matter that I played football, it doesn't matter that I got famous, it doesn't matter that I was in a hundred movies, it doesn't matter, none of it matters. I can't breathe. I keep my hand up like a fucking useless Statue of Liberty, even though I'm alone and no one can help me and the water's getting deeper and colder and I'm falling and I'm drowning . . .

And every time, every fucking time it happened, when I'd given up and the water was seeping into my lungs and I was falling further and further, it was then that a hand broke through the surface of the water – was it a few feet above me, or miles, I couldn't tell? – and reached down to grab me. The grip was firm, but kind; the hand first grasped my wrist so that I was safe, then it slipped into my hand, fingers entwined, the softest, most beautiful feeling you can imagine, soft skin but safe, making me safe, and the hand would pull, pulling me up towards the light, up towards air.

It was Tans. It was always Tans. My beautiful, sweet, funny, kind, tough, modest, loving Tanya. When I was at my lowest, or when I had totally fucked up again, or when things had gone so wrong and I'd let everyone down – when I was drowning, she'd always reach down to grab me, pulling me to safety.

10

You have no idea how it felt . . . or maybe you do. Maybe you've got someone in your life who pulls you out of the deepest waters. I hope you do. I did, for 27 amazing years. Tanya was my lifeguard when I got stupid and swam too deep, or when the black dog of anger threw me into rip tides of rage.

Now, though, when I reach up, no hand ever comes. I have to get out of this alone. I still stretch out my arm, up, up towards the light, hoping that someone will grab me and pull me above the surface. But no. The hand never comes, not anymore. I'm trying not to drown, here.

I'm really trying not to drown.

I've told a lot of people through the years that I think Tans was saved with her heart transplant in order to save me. I don't mean that in an arrogant way. What I mean is, there had to be a reason why she survived her heart collapsing, why they found a heart for her (in Germany, of all places), and there had to be a reason we ended up living next door to each other without knowing it – there had to be a reason for all the coincidences. Because it's such a huge thing, this love we had. I've always believed in premonitions and I think there's something out there that brought us together and kept us together for nearly three decades.

Even how we met – 40 years ago – was a fluke.

1

SUN SPORTS SUNDAYS

If you guessed I've always been a bit of a scallywag, then you'd have guessed right. In fact, I was acting up when I first met a beautiful girl called Tanya Lamont.

We both grew up in Watford: me, on the edge of a council estate, Tanya right bang in the middle of one – 75 Gaddesden Crescent.

Tanya Lamont's childhood was secure and happy.

She was born on Thursday 14 April 1966 into an evening blanketed with a late-season, thick snow. The flakes fell all day across southern England, and by the time Tanya was born – 10.15 p.m. – 15 centimetres of the white stuff had settled across Watford.

In those days, first children were delivered in hospital, an honour bestowed on Tans' elder brother, Shane, but when a second child was ready to appear, you had it at home, no questions asked. Her mum, Maureen, had been to the doctor that morning before the snow had gotten heavy and he'd told her she was in labour; the midwife arrived at their house on Ganders Ash in Watford that evening at 9.30.

Lou, Tans' dad, was watching football on *Sportsview* on the telly in the living room. Forty-five minutes later his daughter was born in the adjoining dining room, was wrapped in a blanket and handed to him. She was a big baby, 8 pounds 12 ounces. Maureen and Lou hadn't known what the gender would be, but quickly landed on Tanya for a name. The footie over, Lou watched the boxing with his newborn in his arms.

In June that year, the growing family moved to Gaddesden Crescent and by the start of 1967 Tanya Lamont was already walking. Shane, three years older, adored his sister, and she adored him right back. Lou and Maureen and Shane and Tanya were an unusually close family and they'd stay that way for the rest of Tanya's life.

It quickly became apparent that Tanya was a special and very interesting child. Shane remembers her sitting in the coal bunker out the back of their house with just her nappy on, merrily chewing on hunks of anthracite. When the coalman arrived, someone in the family would have to run out to check Tanya wasn't in there before he dumped the coal. Sometimes her mum would find her covered in soot, black all over, happy as Larry.

Little Tanya Lamont had about her a kind of magic; she was kind and inquisitive, and fearless, and strikingly beautiful; she wore a leotard non-stop so that she could practise her gymnastics at a moment's notice. She'd do backward somersaults in the living room and, as they grew older, she and her friends would use the low walls on the Gaddesden estate as a balance beam.

Gaddesden was one of those places where everyone knew everyone else and everyone looked out for everyone else. All the houses had three bedrooms, and everyone had a bunch of kids. To her dying day, Tanya stayed friends with many members of her group of friends from the Gaddesden estate – the Gadd Gang, as it was known. The Gadd Gang would do plays and skits and pantomimes, and make Shane be the stagehand. Tanya would dress up in her mother's clothes (Shane is adamant he wasn't made to do the same!).

Gaddesden Crescent was filled with kind people who would look out for each other's kids; in fact, it was a fine place to be born, in the middle of Britain, in the middle of the Swinging Sixties, and just ten weeks before England won the World Cup.

At five years old, Tanya happily toddled off to Lea Farm Infant School – Maureen and Lou waved her off and she barely looked back. She loved school; the place really was built on an old farm (back when it was a farm Maureen and her friends used to hop the fence and nick the eggs) and was a lovely place to go every day. Tanya was a good student and was such a talented young actress that she was picked to be in all the plays – she was Tinkerbell in *Peter Pan*, and, somehow, Cleopatra.

But what really stood out about Tans from a very early age was her ability to love and to love unconditionally. If Tanya loved you – and I was lucky enough to experience this for nearly three decades – then she held back nothing. Her mum describes her as having some sort of 'flair', too, a specialness that everyone noticed. She wasn't a spiritual person, but she was certainly different from the other girls. She was very perceptive – maybe it was her Irish background, sprinkling some faerie dust on her. Whatever it was, that fierceness of love never left her.

The first person outside of Lou, Maureen, and Shane on whom she bestowed this love was Lou's dad, Grandad Tommy. By all reports, Tommy was a very wise man, very steady. A veteran of the Second World War, Tommy Lamont had survived everything Hitler had thrown at him before returning to his hometown of Ballymoney, Northern Ireland. In the late forties, Tommy, his wife Ella and their only child, Lou, had relocated to Ganders Ash in Watford to work at the nearby De Havilland factory (which is now the Warner Bros. studios in Leavesden) and by the time Tanya came along, Lou's Irish accent was fading.

Tanya got a lot of her character from her Grandad Tommy. He was a very genuine man, and they adored each other. But tragedy was to strike. One day in 1978, Ella had waved Tommy off to work from their house on Ganders Ash, but before he'd even reached High Road, the next street over, Tommy Lamont had fallen face first into the pavement; he'd had a massive and fatal heart attack at the age of 69. Tanya was 12 and inconsolable. The heart of someone so close to her had failed; before another decade had passed, her own was to fail, too.

But before tragedy struck, a happy 1960s had quietly

turned into a happy 1970s. Like so many families in the 1970s, the Lamonts looked forward to their week (and later their fortnight) by the sea each summer. They'd picked a town called St Osyth, a few miles west of Clacton-on-Sea. There, in a caravan on the Bel Air Chalet Estate, Maureen and her sister and the kids played on the beach by day, and at night they'd all go to the clubhouse where 50 pence would get the ladies a half pint of lager and the kids a bottle of pop. One year, a lovely hippy-dippy family showed up next door to the Lamonts and Tans, ever the seeker, became very close to them, holding deep conversations about spiritual things. They taught her to meditate and chant and gave her a copy of the New Age classic, *Jonathan Livingston Seagull*.

But Tans was also obsessed, like so many other teens and pre-teens, by matters less spiritual, like David Cassidy, and like so many young girls, horses.

At the time, there were TV shows on like *White Horses* and *Black Beauty*, and Tans never missed them. Tanya had this dream of having her own horse and riding it through Montana, as free as could be – although through Garston Park and up the hill into the long grass would have to do. She always thought she was in an episode of *Little House on the Prairie*. The sun was her thing; a sunny, spring day was her idea of heaven.

And then her dad became her superhero when he brought Persephone home on her twelfth birthday.

Persephone was a big horse for a 12-year-old – at least 15 hands. Tanya's dad had done a bit of this and a bit of that and had gotten the money together to make his daughter's greatest dream come true. Tans couldn't believe her eyes; she didn't sleep for days after the horse showed up, and from that day on her family barely saw her – she was always off with Persephone, grooming, feeding, mucking out, and riding riding riding.

Her dad had organized a spot up the road in a field to graze the beast, but that didn't stop Tanya riding it down Gaddesden Crescent whenever she could. The neighbours would go potty – Mr Kimba across the road from number 75, who was known locally as a right case – or, as Maureen once described him, 'a miserable old bugger' – was particularly unhappy about this massive beast wandering down the centre of his street and once chased her with his walking stick right across Garston Park. But nothing, not even an angry old dodderer, stopped Tanya riding Persephone wherever she wanted.

She'd even ride it along the A405; I can't imagine what car drivers thought when they saw this young girl on top of this big horse on the North Orbital, going past the Three Horseshoes and into Garston Park. It can't have been legal, but then, I knew Tanya – when she had something in her mind, she did it, and that was that.

After about six months of riding, the summer of 1978 arrived, and Tanya and Persephone were inseparable. While most people were lining up to see *Grease*, *Saturday Night Fever* or *Close Encounters of the Third Kind*, Tanya was astride Persephone in the narrow streets of Watford. Except for one afternoon, when Tanya briefly went missing and Persephone got stuck in Maureen's kitchen.

Tanya had, yet again, and in the face of the neighbours' complaints, ridden Persephone like a Commanche to 75 Gaddesden Crescent so her friends could coo and stroke and maybe get a ride on the huge brute. Tanya had parked Persephone in the back garden, where the sweet thing decided to do its bit and nibble the long grass down to an acceptable length, as horses will (she may or may not have also eaten some roses from the next door's garden). Tanya went off to fetch her friends, at which point Maureen thought it would be a good idea to offer the animal a carrot to distract her from the roses. There was a big bag of them just inside the kitchen, so Tanya's mum reached in and got her the veg – but Persephone, clearly with an eye for the main chance, swallowed the carrot sharpish and decided to head up the two big concrete steps and into the kitchen for the rest of the bag.

At which point, Mrs Maureen Lamont had a 15-hand Arabian horse in her kitchen. And no daughter in sight.

Horses do what horses want, especially when they're stuck in a kitchen in Watford. The poor thing's head pretty much reached the ceiling, and Maureen, and Shane, who had now appeared from the living room, had no idea how to get the horse back out into the garden. There was no turning the thing around – horses don't like reverse gear all that much – and the two big concrete steps were two steps too far for the nag. And, even without that impediment, there was still the little matter of neither Shane nor his mum knowing the correct clucks to make reverse happen.

Tanya might have known, but Tanya was nowhere to be found.

It was then Shane had the brilliant idea that instead of trying to *reverse* the horse, maybe it made sense to lead it through the house by the nose and out the front door. The horse, now filled with a bag of carrots, didn't seem to mind – but to repeat, *with the horse now filled with carrots,* time was of the essence, because any moment Persephone might be donating a heap of something to grouchy Mrs Nicell next door for what was left of her roses.

There was no time to waste – Shane held a carrot and his mum pushed the horse's arse. At first, Persephone seemed perfectly comfortable in the kitchen and refused to budge. Shane swung the carrot to and fro and Maureen heaved from the rear. Eventually, the horse reluctantly started to move, slowly and heavily through the tight hallway towards the closed front door. Shane got it open just as the animal was about to get stuck near the stairs. There, lo and behold, on the other side of the now-opened front door, stood Roger, the milkman, who was at that moment delivering two pints and a bottle of pop.

Being a British milkman, Roger must have seen everything at least once, and probably prided himself, as all British milkmen do, on not being impressed by anything. Without so much as a raised eyebrow, Roger took in the scene – a pimply 16-year old boy waving a carrot, behind which a 15-hand Arabian loomed, behind which a red-faced woman was pushing and clucking fit to burst – and merely said 'Alright there, Mrs.' (Referring, presumably, to

Maureen Lamont, not Persephone.) With that, Roger put down the pints, turned on his heel, and sauntered back to his electric milk truck, without another word or even a look back.

With the milkman out of the way, Shane and his mum managed to squeeze the horse out through the door and onto the path, where it knocked over the pints before it resumed grazing, this time on the front lawn. Eventually, Tanya arrived back with her friends, none the wiser, and ready to continue the most magical summer of her young life.

Later that magical summer, Persephone made another visit to Maureen's kitchen – because once you invite a horse into a kitchen, it's pretty much going to believe the invitation is an open one. Again, carrots, but this time, a heaping pile of leavings, too, right by the fridge. And again, no reverse gear available, so off down the hallway towards the front door, pausing only to stick its head into the living room in case there were carrots in there, too. There were no carrots, only a visiting TV repair man, who had heard the clatter of hooves and had looked up just in time to see Persephone's head appear in the doorway.

'Fucking hell!' he shouted in abject fear, proving, if further proof was needed, that if you ever find yourself in a tight spot and you need someone to stay calm and back you up, pick the milkman, not the TV repairman.

Summer 1978 was also when I met Tanya Lamont for the first time.

I went to a school that's no longer there – Langleybury, a big old comprehensive which used to be in the north-west corner of Watford; she went to the Francis Combe Academy, about three miles east of Langleybury. But it could have been a million miles away to be honest: ours was known as the 'prison on the hill'. It was so unlikely that the two of us would ever have met – literal worlds apart – that is, until fate threw us together in Watford's Whippendell Woods.

On weekends I'd sometimes go to a rec centre called Sun Postal Sports and Social Club. Right on the edge of Whippendell Woods, Sun Sports, as we called it, had a cricket pitch and a football field and a bar and a meeting hall and all that – the kind of place people go to have their weddings. We kids would hang out there and run around sometimes, climb trees, all the usual things kids do while their parents are busy playing cricket or having a drink.

One weekend, when I was about 13, I'd gone to Sun Sports with my mate Russell and a few other friends and, unbeknownst to me, Tans – who was about 12 – was there with a couple of her friends, as one of their dads was in the cricket team. The two groups were messing around together, climbing trees and all that, and I can remember her so vividly, still, to this very day: long hair, beautiful thick eyebrows, kind smile, reserved but confident. But even then, I knew she was so far out my league that it was like she was from a different planet.

So, faced with a girl who I knew would never waste an

ounce of interest on me, I did what any self-respecting 13-year-old boy thinking about girls for pretty much the first time would do – I started showing off. Behind the clubhouse at Sun Sports there was a fenced-off area filled with crates of beer and pop and at some point Tanya Lamont must have said she wanted a drink because, before anyone could stop me, I'd climbed over the fence and nicked her a can of Tizer, and that was it.

(On the *Keith Barret Show* in 2005, Tans told Rob Brydon a bit of a different story: 'Vin had just broken into the bar,' she said, 'climbed over a fence; all the bottles of beer had tar on, so he was smashing the beers and trying to drink them . . . Then he walked round the corner and I said to my friend, "Oh, who's that boy?"'

This is just another of the reasons my heart is broken – I can't compare stories with her any more. I either stole her a can of pop, or I was breaking the tops off beer bottles. I guess I'll never know.)

I didn't know it then – how could I? – but that was the start of the most important thing that ever happened to me. Forget playing for Wimbledon or *Lock Stock* or Dave Bassett or Guy Ritchie. Yes, those things have given me an amazing life, and I'm grateful for all of them – but I owe the most crucial relationship of my life to Sun Sports and the makers of Tizer (or perhaps bottles of beer).

I don't remember a single thing we said to each other, but I still remember trying to be all cocky. I wonder what she saw back then . . . I've thought since that in my worst moments, Tans has always been able to see past the fights and the bullshit and the bad publicity and the stupid things I've done, to the 13-year-old in me, the kid *before* the hurt and the fame and the drink kicked in.

Because I may have half-inched a Tizer, but that was as bad as it ever got back then. I honestly wouldn't even nick someone's apple off a tree. I knew it was wrong. To my mind, there are 'rogues' – lads that'll have a fight and things like that – and then there are slippery fuckers who are thieves and deceitful. I was never that. That just wasn't my game. If the football went on the school roof, ten lads might go up there to get the ball, no problem, but the one time I went, I'd get caught. That was me.

But other than the Tizer incident, to impress Tans, I was never a thief. Well, except once, and it was another crucial moment in my young life.

When I was about seven years old, I found out that my dad kept a stash of cash in his office, in a drawer. For days I fought the urge to take some, but in the end my desire to be popular with my mates took over and I started to pinch a few tenners here and there to buy sweets for everyone. Eventually, my parents noticed the loss and called the police; it didn't take long for two and two to be put together, as both my teacher at primary school and the local sweetshop owner had noticed I was suddenly awash with moolah.

My dad's reaction still haunts me; his disappointment was matched by a hiding he gave me that I can still feel. I was also grounded for the entire summer; it was 1972, and while everyone else was out playing footy, I was locked in like a skinhead Rapunzel watching the Munich Olympics (I still hate the javelin).

What happened that summer stuck with me; I knew what I'd done was all wrong, and I was never tempted to thieve again. Instead, I got up to other kinds of mischief. This, for example: both of the school buses – the one for Langleybury and the one for Francis Combe – used to park behind each other up in Bedmond where we lived. Some mornings, just for a change, I'd get on the Francis Combe bus instead of the Langleybury one and go into the wrong school. I had two good mates, Mark and Paul, who went to Francis Combe, and I'd pretend I was their cousin from Devon, even though I had a Watford accent. I'd spend the day there, going to class with them and playing football.

I don't remember if I saw Tans at Francis Combe or not, or if she saw me.

I can't ask her now. I can't ask her anything.

Despite me stealing money from him, in my early years my dad and I were really good – we'd go fishing and shooting together, and we were actually a close family. When I was about seven, we moved from Newhouse Crescent, north of Watford, to Lower Paddock Road in Oxhey, south of Watford centre. At around that time, my younger sister, Ann, had had a bone marrow transplant, and the experience had drawn us all together . . . or so I thought.

The reality would prove to be much darker.

As a kid you never think your parents would ever split up, even when they're fighting a lot. A kid's view of the world

25

is pretty simple: Mum and Dad and siblings are there, you go to school and see your friends; sometimes there's fun, sometimes you're in trouble, sometimes everything's OK. I played football, of course – the fields were right behind my house – we traded and banged marbles, and we rode bikes around Oxhey Green and Attenborough Fields. Sometimes when we got a bit daring we'd go as far as Merry Hill Wood. For a few years it was idyllic; I had a very happy childhood, all told.

And then Dad decided we had to move to Bedmond, near Hemel Hempstead. Though it was only eight miles away, we might as well have been moving to the moon. I was leaving all my friends and my school, and even though we were heading to a much better house, I freaked out. I did everything I could to stop the move – I think I even took a pair of scissors to some curtains. But Mum and Dad weren't having it, and they outlasted my upset.

But once again I was saved by something I didn't understand. Around that time, I had a dream about a football pitch. In the dream there was a main road, and a little lane, and a gap in the green plastic fence, and a bollard stopping cars getting in, and it was on the left – I can still see it, clear as day: the little football pitch on the left of my dream.

On my first day in Bedmond, imagine my amazement when dad sent me out to explore and I found the exact football field from my dream, across Bedmond Road, then right on Tom's Lane. Walking along, on the left I saw the chain-link fence, and the bollard, and the wide-open expanse of green, and the posts and nets – exactly the same as the dream I'd had – and I think I knew then I'd be alright.

2

WATFORD BOYS

And I *was* alright, until I wasn't.

I got picked by Watford Boys when I was about 12 years old and ended up captaining them. I played alongside a bunch of good players, too, including Nigel Callaghan, who'd go on to feature in Watford's 1984 Cup Final team. But something was going on at home that put the kibosh on my teen years: my parents were breaking up, and it wasn't pretty.

Luckily for me, during the days I was out playing football all the time, and when I wasn't playing, I was watching – Watford had even given me a pass to get into any game I wanted. Everyone in the family had been so proud of me. I was good back then, head and shoulders – both physically, and skills-wise – over the other lads.

It was in my blood I suppose. I was born across the street from Vicarage Road, in the old Shrodell's Hospital, and the second I was born my dad picked me up, took me to the window – I was maybe one minute old, apparently – and, pointing at the stadium, he said, 'You'll play there one day.'

My grandad was a staunch Watford supporter, all my uncles were too, and I still am. We all loved the football club.

When I was growing up, we travelled all over the country to watch them. And don't forget what happened to that club: in 1977 we were bottom of the league – I don't mean bottom of the old First Division, I mean the bottom of ALL the leagues, propping up the old Fourth Division. But lifelong fan Elton John came aboard and pumped some money in – he had been the chairman for a year when he signed up Graham Taylor to manage us.

Jump forward to five games into the 1982–83 season and we were top of the league – and I don't mean the old Fourth Division, I mean the top of the old First Division. In fact, in the fourth game of that season, we'd beaten Sunderland 8–0. What a ride – in five years we'd gone from the worst to the best!

We'd all travel to Nottingham Forest, who were a top team then, and Liverpool, and West Ham, and Man United, and Southampton – I remember us beating them lot 7–1 in the League Cup in 1980 (we'd been one–nil down at half time – talk about a game of two halves!). And Elton? He said in his autobiography that Watford might have saved his life. He wrote:

> I was chairman throughout the worst period of my life: years of addiction and unhappiness, failed relationships, bad business deals, court cases, unending turmoil. Through all of that, Watford were a constant source of happiness to me . . . For obvious reasons,

there are chunks of the eighties I have no recollection of – but every Watford game I saw is permanently etched on my memory.

What a guy.

So, just like Elton, Watford is in my blood, in my case from the second I started screaming in the bassinet at Shrodell's.

But though in my early teen years the days were filled with footy, the nights were terrible.

Dad had built us the house in Bedmond, and he'd put his heart into it, but my parents weren't getting along – at all. At night I'd sneak into my sister Ann's room to comfort her as they raged at each other into the wee hours; me and my sister would hug each other, praying the screaming and carrying on would soon stop. And it wasn't as if me and Ann really got along all that well. It shows, though, how kids often try to make the best of everything. It still hurts that we were forced to care about each other like that; it still feels unfair and it left me less and less certain of people, and more and more wary – and angry.

I'd always been a sweet enough kid; I messed around, yes, but I wasn't angry deep down, not at all. I was a scally, not a nutter. But something about listening all those nights to the angry fights, and the fact that me and my sister were left to fend for ourselves upstairs . . . Adult arguments are terrifying for kids, who feel out of control, scared, unable to process the complicated hurts they can hear being aired by the two people they most need to be solid and secure.

What I'm saying is, that 13-year-old that Tanya Lamont met at Sun Sports? He was getting harried by hurt into a much tougher proposition. I'm actually a sensitive little kid at heart; I'm not afraid to admit that. Talking so much about losing Tanya and being emotional about it in public has surprised some people I think; but the truth is that I've always been emotional. So hearing my parents' marriage disintegrate was murder for me; it left me empty and unable to focus on football. Football? Actually, who cared? Ann and I had been up all night clinging on for dear life – so what if I missed some training here and there? Even when I did make it to training, my mind wasn't fully on it.

The end came when I was 16 years old.

Things at home got really terrible. A friend of my mum's had shown up at our house and admitted that, years before, she'd slept with my dad. I have no idea to this day why that woman thought she needed to get that off her chest, but she did, and it only deepened the disaster that was home. Soon after, Mum's friends showed up to help her move out. I screamed at them, but it was no use. She went off to live in the nursing home where she worked and Dad had to sell the house he'd built to pay her.

Which left Ann and me adrift. I was mad at both my parents, but I think especially at my mum. Dad did a good job of making her the monster – understandable, but only half the story. I was still trying to get to football practices, but it was a losing battle.

One day, I was pulled into the office by Tom Walley, the legendary coach at Watford, and Bertie Mee, himself a legend from his ten years managing the Arsenal (including during the League and Cup double year of 1971). Mee was Graham Taylor's assistant and head of scouting, meaning he basically ran the Watford youth team. When I knew him, he was in his sixties, but still as sharp as ever, a real football man.

This was the time that I was either going to be signed on real apprenticeship forms, or I was done. I thought I had a shot but Tom Walley and Bertie Mee had called me in to tell me they were letting me go. One of their reasons was that I wasn't big enough – at the time, Watford seemed obsessed with the size of their players and for some reason they thought I was too small – which is pretty funny, given how my career panned out as a well-built Mr Hard Man. But at the time they were adamant.

That wasn't the worst bit, though. No, what Mee said to me cut me to the bone. It's hard to hear terrible news from anyone but especially a legend – and even more so because he couldn't really have known how wrong he was, and how lacking in understanding of what I was going through.

'You treat life as a joke,' Mee said. He also said that maybe Spurs or Coventry were interested, but his comment about treating life as a joke really hurt and shut me down for good. He couldn't have known what I was going through at home, I suppose, but the reality was that life wasn't much of a joke, that was for sure.

I don't hate Bertie Mee, but I think it's a good lesson in being careful what you say to people, especially young people. You can never know what someone's going through.

I've found this out a lot since Tans died. If it looks like someone is finding life to be too much of a joke, chances are something else is going on under the surface.

At about the same time, though, thank god, there was something funny happening elsewhere – Tanya's dad, Lou, was somewhere in Watford hitting a donkey's cock with a stick.

What had happened was that the donkey – a field-mate to Persephone – had taken a liking to the horse and whenever possible would attempt an amorous mounting, despite the difference in size and, let's be honest, species. Clearly the donkey was hankering after giving the world one more mule – all reports suggest that, and here I quote Tans' mum, Maureen, 'His thing used to hang all the way to the ground; it was shocking.' Persephone had no such plans, so it seems. Shane adds to the reminiscences with a memorable phrase: 'My dad,' Shane says, 'had to regularly beat the donkey's dongle with a stick.'

'That bloody donkey again,' Lou would say. Eventually, Persephone got wise to the donkey and would chase it away, but not before the donkey bit a chunk out of Persephone's rear. Something had to give, and Tanya's mind had moved to other things in any case, as 16-year-olds' minds will, and Persephone was sold.

Gaddesden Crescent would never be the same. And I imagine the donkey never got over it, either.

As for me? I was done too; for the next three years, I didn't kick a ball in anger. I had no one on my side; my dad had had to sell the house he'd built for us at Woodlands to pay mum and he was in a new relationship; Mum was living in the nursing home where she worked and had someone new too. I'd see her once in a while, but I hated it; it didn't feel right, and Dad had a lot of anger towards her then too, which poisoned me against her for a while. It seems that there wasn't any room left for me in anyone's life; they all had their own shit to deal with. And Watford Boys had let me go – so what, right?

I was still living with my dad, but I was spending a lot of time with a local gamekeeper, Neil Robinson, and his 'wife' Andrea. (Dad had actually hired them to work on his property – he ran a local shoot – on the old-fashioned condition that they be married, which was pretty rich coming from a guy who was getting divorced. Neil and Andrea had worn rings to the interview, but it was clear to anyone with half a brain that there was no way they were married, though they eventually sneaked off to get wed and no one was any the wiser.) But Dad started to get jealous that I was spending a lot of time with Neil – I think he felt Neil was looking out for me in ways that he couldn't and he was right – Neil *was* like a father figure when I needed one. For my part, I played it up a bit with Dad; I was cheeky about it as I knew it needled him and, honestly, I was deep down so hurt by everything that I don't think I cared if I upset him.

Eventually, Dad and Neil had a huge argument about the situation. I took Neil's side, as ever, and that might have been the end of it . . . but Dad wasn't done. Right there and then he hauled off and gave me a right-hander, standing on our doorstep, knocking me through the sliding door and right back into the house.

It was the first time he'd hit me since I'd stolen that money when I was seven, but this was different. I was 16. Watford had let me go. I had quit school without sitting a single exam and I was either on the dole or doing hod-carrying work. My parents were split, I felt alone in the world and my dad had just smacked me right across my face. So I just walked into our house, my cheek still stinging, put my stuff in black bin liners – my records, my footy medals and some clothes – and walked away.

Neil and Andrea took me in for a while until they set me up with job in the kitchens at Bradfield College near Pangbourne, down in the Chilterns. I was the washer-upper; it sounds like hell I suppose, but it wasn't *all* bad. I had my own room with a single bed, though it was above the kitchen, so everything stank of the cooking. As the pot washer I worked seven till seven, every day – Bradfield is a posh boarding school – but at least I had time off in the afternoon until I had to come back and get ready for the evening meal. I learned quickly to never get to work late, because the pots used to be to the ceiling if I didn't get a good start on them. I suppose I ate OK – I'd scrounge the leftovers of those boys. And what boys they were! The college is known for putting on Greek plays – *in Greek* – and for running a course in the summer on how to improve your bellringing. I wonder what they'd think if they realized Vinnie Jones, the guy who grabbed Gazza by the knackers, used to work there, cleaning their pots and pans.

Needless to say, I only stuck it out for a year. I'm amazed I did that long to be honest. Greek and bellringing? Whatever.

I haven't lived under the same roof as my dad since. Some days I can still feel that smack. Tans was always so good about helping me forgive him, for seeing his side, for making just the right excuses for the old fella, and for my mum, too. She did that for everyone.

Tans also had a very special bond with my mother, whose early life was tragic. When she was very young, my mum was taking one of her younger sisters to school and they were standing on the side of the road waiting to cross. One of their little friends waved across to them and my mum's sister pulled out of my mum's hand and ran into the street where she was hit by a lorry and killed. My mum's mum, my grandmother, never forgave my mum; in fact, she put her in a home soon after. Tans knew all this and, as ever, she loved an underdog. Knowing what my mum had gone through helped her understand me, too. Tans would say, 'Vin is a beautiful boy, very complex.' She knew all of the parts that created me, all of the different sides of how I was raised, even when it was hurtful to me, and I couldn't see past the pain my parents had caused.

I don't know how she was so loving, but I was so grateful she helped me see the good in people. That's something I think about when the grief is deep – not just what I lost when she went, but all the things I gained by just knowing her. I think trying to focus on that every day will help me get through it. She was always emotionally making the bed for everyone – making it comfortable, better, with corners that hold you tight.

So it's no surprise to me that in her life, she was the proud owner of not just one but two hearts.

3

THE STOLEN SUZUKI

Eventually I ended up back nearer home, working on building sites when I wasn't on the dole. At the time I was riding around on a little Suzuki motorbike. I don't think I even owned it; some lad at work had given it to me and I was to pay him when I got my wages. I remember clearly that there was no key – you had to start it with a screwdriver – so who knows if my mate owned it either. But it got me around, and that's all that mattered.

One night, when I was about 18 years old, I rode the bike to a pub called the Three Horseshoes in Garston, in the north end of Watford. And who should be there but Tanya Lamont? I hadn't seen her since Sun Sports, but in the intervening few years she'd gotten even more beautiful, if such a thing was possible. I'd never seen anyone with longer, more gorgeous hair and her smile was so wide . . . That night, in that pub, it was like there was no one there except her; I couldn't take my eyes off her. Fortunately, she noticed me too and said hello, calling me, as she always did back then, Vincent. We got to talking and I told her about leaving home and going away to the Chilterns and the problems with my dad and what had happened with Watford, and she was so sweet about it all. I could have talked to her all night.

At the time she was still living with her parents in Gaddesden Crescent, which was only a five-minute walk away, straight across the Kingsway and through Garston Park. She told me she was allowed down the pub, but she had to be home before her dad got in. He was very protective and she, in turn, adored him. So even though it was much earlier than I was used to leaving a pub, it was the least I could do to offer to walk her home, so that's what I did.

By the time we got to Gaddesden Crescent – five, six minutes later – I was back in love. There was no one like her and never had been. I was only 18 years old, but I knew she was the one for me. And yet, she was so out of my orbit I was certain that there was no way she could ever love me back. I was just a lad trying to get my head above water; I was flitting from couch to couch, holding down this job, that job, the other. My parents had split, I was working here and there, but I wasn't making much of myself. I'd been at a posh school washing pots and pans and trying to get the sound of fucking bellringing out of my head. My football career had gone south and I really had no prospects. But this young woman, unlocking the front door to 75 Gaddesden Crescent ... she was something else. She had poise, and she was smart and beautiful, and she was going to be something.

What was I going to do? She was everything, even then.

Suddenly, I was in her kitchen and Maureen was making a pot of tea and I couldn't believe I was in Tanya Lamont's house, with her. I was so punching above my weight – and that's a feeling I had until the day she died. I had the feeling that night for certain as I chatted with her mother and Tanya before her dad got home, the three of us sitting around their Formica kitchen table, the one with the red and white checkers.

I was determined to do everything right; I was already a better person just by being in the same room as her. I wasn't acting all Jack-the-Lad; I was respectful, just grateful to be there. Her mum was so nice to me too – they both treated me with respect and warmth. But I knew I shouldn't overstay my welcome – her dad was due home any minute – so I made my excuses, gave Tanya the slightest peck on the cheek and headed out the back door.

I left the house on cloud nine. The five minutes back to the Three Horseshoes took a millisecond. All I could think of was the softness of her cheek as I'd kissed her goodnight.

But things just never went right for me back then. I felt like a big dark cloud followed me around. I still had to pick up my Suzuki at the pub, but when I got there it was nearly midnight and the place was closed up. Worse: where my motorbike had been, now there was just the stupid, huge helmet I'd wear, sitting on the front step of the pub.

Nicked.

It was the first time something of mine had been stolen and I needed that bike to get around, back and forth to work and all that. I was fuming and freaking out. Now I was stuck in Garston with no ride to whichever couch I was staying on that night, and I hadn't even paid for the thing yet. What the hell was I going to do?

It was late enough that there wasn't much traffic about and above the sound of the odd truck on the Kingsway, somewhere in the distance I could hear a high-pitched whine, like the sound of a cheap motorcycle. On a hunch, I picked up my helmet and followed the sound until I got to Garston Park. Once there, it was obvious what was happening. I thought, 'You're fucking joking.' In the dimly lit park, I could make out a few lads who'd been hanging out with Tans and her mates in the pub earlier – now, they were joyriding the Suzuki up and down, hooting and shouting and laughing and doing wheelies and all that.

I wasn't having it. Sneaking behind a tree, I waited for the bike to get closer, and as it passed, I stepped out and swung my helmet at the kid on my bike. Bosh – down he goes like a ton of bricks, the bike toppling over and stalling. I think he was more startled than hurt; he quickly jumped up and ran and all of his mates ran off too, leaving me with a banged-up, keyless Suzuki and a horrible feeling in the pit of my stomach. Not because they'd nicked my bike, though that had been bad enough. What I felt then was that I'd maybe been set up by Tanya Lamont. Perhaps she'd only agreed to let me walk her home so that her mates could steal my bike and have a drunken ride around Garston Park.

All my insecurities came flooding back, there in the dark park with my motorcycle on the ground. My demons, which I fought and fought, showed up once again; the big cloud got darker, deeper. All my trust in people had been shattered by what had happened at home, so I was able to see betrayal everywhere I looked.

Would Tanya set me up like that? Well, of course she would; it wasn't that she was *bad*, it was just that I didn't register in her life, and certainly not in her heart. I was several thousand miles from being at her level, so of course she'd help her *real* friends pinch my motorbike. She was just a beautiful decoy.

I was underwater and she was up there on the surface, swimming through life.

Tans was always the other side of the M1 from me; there was no way across. And what happened in May 1984 proved it, though I wasn't to know it at the time.

On 19 May 1984, my beloved Watford ran out at Wembley to play Everton in the F.A. Cup Final. This was the great Graham Taylor-led team featuring Nigel Callaghan, Mo Johnston and John Barnes. That said, the Everton team weren't bad that day, either – Neville Southall in goal, Gary Stevens and Trevor Steven confusing commentators up and down the country, Peter Reid in midfield and Graeme Sharp, Adrian Heath and Andy Gray up front.

Playing centre back that day for Watford was Steve Terry – remember him? He always wore a big white sticky bandage on his forehead. He'd first cut his head badly in an aerial duel with Justin Fashanu against Norwich in the early eighties (I would go on to be mates with Justin's brother, John). In those days, there was no concussion protocol –

you got stitched up and sent back out. That's what had happened to Steve; they patched him up, sent him back on but, because he was a tall centre back, he'd of course have to head the ball at some point – when he did so, it opened up the wound all over again. Ridiculous. After that, he wore the big plaster on his head during games to stop the old wound rupturing.

But despite all that, Steve Terry made quite the career for himself at Watford. I, on the other hand, had screwed it up completely.

On the day of the Cup Final I was 19 years old; I wasn't playing football, I was just Vinnie Jones, working-class guy with no real prospects, doing this, that and the other. Tanya Lamont? No idea. After the Suzuki incident I'd accused her of setting me up and we'd fallen out. And it hadn't helped that someone told her I was claiming we'd had a snog on the way home (I didn't tell anyone that – it wasn't true for a start, but also I would never brag about such a thing in any case). But we lost contact once again, and I figured that was it forever.

When I got let go from Watford, Nigel Callaghan had got taken on, and now he was in the first team and getting ready to play in the Cup final. Nigel was from Garston – right across the street from the Three Horseshoes, if you need one more coincidence. Nigel was a good lad and had slung a couple of Cup Final tickets to my mate Russell, who – if you remember – had been with me the day at Sun Sports when I'd first met Tanya Lamont. Russell knew I'd been a Watford fan all my life and that I was on my arse at the time and he offered me the second ticket. Cup Final tickets were like gold dust in those days; Wembley held 100,000 people (and then some), but you were still really lucky if you could get a ticket. There was no secondary online market in those days; it was either a tout or nowt.

It was a gorgeous, early summer day in north London. My beloved Watford had made it to the Cup Final for the first time in their history and everywhere we looked we saw a sea of gold scarves. It seemed like the whole town had shown up. Elton John had brought some razzmatazz to the club for sure, but they were also a really good team (they'd finished second in the league behind Liverpool a year earlier). We were all pinching ourselves that we'd made it to Wembley . . . and I couldn't help thinking that I could have been in that team if things had been different. Then again, it was a bit like how I felt about Tanya Lamont; she was also a million miles from me, so there was no point harbouring too much of an upset about it.

But just as I was thinking about how life had gone south, Tanya was right in front of me, though I had no idea.

Russell and I were standing on Wembley Way, looking to cross the road to head into the stadium, when a big bus draped in Watford colours came along. Some copper stopped us – threw his arm right across us – as the bus passed. It couldn't have been the team bus as the players had been in Wembley for a while, probably, warming up and doing that poncy walkabout before the game. I looked at Russell and nodded at the bus, saying, 'players' wives and girlfriends'. I thought nothing more of it.

What I couldn't know was that at that exact moment Tanya Lamont – soon-to-be Tanya Terry – was on the bus, saw me on the pavement and had shouted out my name.

Things had greatly changed for Tanya since I'd walked her home from the Three Horseshoes the night my bike got nicked. She was still living with her parents in Gaddesden Crescent, and it turned out that her next-door neighbour, grouchy Annie Nicell (she of the roses), used to have all the lads from Watford living with her. Graham Taylor had a rule back then that all the players had to live within five miles of Vicarage Road (Gaddesden Crescent is three and a half miles away) so he could keep an eye on everyone and know when they were going out too much (I'm not sure how well I'd have done under Taylor to be honest, at least back then!). He was a stickler, Taylor, big on discipline, which was a difficult task with a bunch of young men. (It was made even more difficult when you remember that Mo Johnston – a man who, according to one article, very much enjoyed the 'flamboyant, high-living champagne lifestyle' – was in that team!) But Taylor's way must have worked – he turned Watford into a really good club.

Anyway, Tanya's neighbour Annie Nicell had John Barnes, Steve Terry and Kenny Jackett all living with her until they made it to the first team and started earning enough money to get their own places. (It didn't come soon enough, apparently: Mrs Nicell fed the lads such inedible mashed potatoes that they used to secrete them in flower pots up and down Gaddesden Crescent.)

Things being how they are, these lads ended up meeting

Tanya and all her friends. One day, a visitor had arrived to see Shane and Tanya, whose job it was every day to wash up after the evening meal, had gone to the front door in her bright yellow Marigolds. As she opened the door, she saw Steve Terry arriving at Annie Nicell's, and shouted hello; they proceeded to chat for a while outside, though Tans never took her rubber gloves off. It didn't seem to dissuade him, though – by 1984 Tanya Lamont and Steve Terry were dating.

Cut to Cup Final day – Tanya is on the wives and girl-friends' bus and clocks me being held back by the copper on the pavement as the coach passes. According to what she told me much later, she ran to the window and shouted my name. She'd probably seen my hair before she'd seen me – back then I had a big old shock of curly hair, a huge thing taking up space above my forehead.

Her friend, Suzy Bicknell (who was dating John Barnes at the time and would subsequently be married to him for a decade), said, 'What are you doing?'

'That's Vincent Jones,' Tanya said.

Suzy was confused, apparently – she probably noticed the way that Tanya had lit up when she'd recognized me, even though she was dating Steve – but soon the bus was out of the traffic and away to the stadium. And I was none the wiser; I just kept on my merry way, went into Wembley, got to my seat and watched Tanya's boyfriend and the rest of his teammates lose to Everton 2–0.

When I'd heard two years later that Tans had married Steve Terry, I thought: 'Yeah, it makes sense – of course she's going out with a pro footballer. Of course she is – she's beautiful and smart and it makes sense.' I didn't even have a little knot in my stomach about it. She was still on the other side of the M1 to me and I couldn't cross. There was too much traffic. It was too dangerous.

No, not dangerous, just impossible. I was ducking and diving, doing a bit of window cleaning, a bit of labouring, I was working at Mitsubishi, temping. Or I was on the dole. But Tans? Married to a First Division footballer who'd already played in the Cup Final, friends with Suzy Barnes and John Barnes – they'd all got on a boat and it was sailing happily down the river.

The M1 is wide, and it never sleeps, and it is impossible to simply run to the other side. I was over *this* side, struggling, stuck outside Wembley, standing on the pavement, being held back; she was on the bus. Being with Tans wasn't even an option.

Even though they'd lost, I remember Watford had a celebration in an open-top bus that ended up at what was then the Watford Harlequin shopping centre. I stood in the huge crowd and quietly said to myself, 'One day I'll play in an F.A. Cup Final.' It was more a dream than a hope.

Until it became a reality, of course.

4

A GANG CALLED CRAZY

When I was about 19, I got a job just south-west of Watford at what was once the Masonic School for Boys on The Avenue in Bushey. My mate Mark Attwood's dad, Pete, was the head groundsman on the property and hired me to be a gardener. It was a beautiful place and my job was to whiz around on one of those huge mowers making everything look like Wembley Stadium.

One day in the summer of 1984, Pete said, 'Do you know the measurements of a football pitch? We've got this team, Wealdstone, coming to do their preseason here.' At the time, Wealdstone were a big deal, at least in non-league football. They were leading the Gola League then (the Gola League became the GM Vauxhall Conference became the Nationwide Conference became the Blue Square Premier and so on – basically, it was the league below the old Division Four) and they would go on to do the League and F.A. Trophy double in 1985.

When the team arrived for their first training session they had a pitch all marked out by yours truly. As they warmed up, I got chatting to Wealdstone's manager at the time, Brian Hall, and I just happened to mention that one of the last big games I'd ever played was here at the school. I said, 'I played for the county.' By this point I was getting back into football a bit – I'd been playing for Bedmond – and, even though I was standing there in my groundsman's overalls, Hall, bless him, told me to bring my gear and join in with training. This was a big deal – at that level, former pros were still plying their trade and an up-and-comer called Stuart Pearce had recently left Wealdstone to join Coventry City (he had played for them for a full five seasons, starting at age 16).

Things went well enough with Wealdstone that I ended up being taken on to the team, though I did manage to fit in a few drunken fights at pubs on away games.

Alcohol . . .

Since Tans died, I've been doing a lot of thinking about how alcohol affected my life.

As I've said, many nights my sister and I would huddle together in her bedroom while downstairs my parents fought out all their hurt. For some people, this might put them off alcohol for life – I met one young lad recently who told me that because his mother was an alcoholic, he has never had a single drink because he associates it with that violent snap that his mother would get.

Sadly, it had the reverse effect on me: I turned to it, and it would make me aggressive. I think that's because I was comfortable with it – I knew how alcohol could breed aggression, and so even though it was deeply painful, I felt at home in that pain; it was just how hurt got released. Even though it's damaging, it was just more comfortable to me to be in the thrall of alcohol. Conflict became something I was used to, because it was every fucking night until three o'clock in the morning. I had found out it was great to have a fight and I was quite good at it. People would say, 'Did you see Jonesy knock him out?' That was all the talk – it had become the weekend sport.

I guess it's all about what side you want to be on. I went to the aggressive, heavy-drinking side because I was comfortable with that side. In my home life there had been drink involved and there were the arguments and everything. For the lad I talked to the other day, well, it worked the other way for him – I wish it had mine.

When I was a young lad and my parents were screaming at each other, I couldn't be as strong as I wanted to be. Alcohol gave me that strength, even when it deeply damaged my life, and more importantly, Tans' life. I wish I could take back the years she knew me as a drinker, but I can't. At least she got the last six years . . . But I'm jumping ahead. I can't help it; I can be telling a story – any story – and the vision of her comes to me and I have to go back to her, to talk to her in my head, to tell her I'm sorry and that I love her and that I hope she was at least a little bit proud of me, even though I could be a right pain in the arse.

Anyway, eventually I got a break into the Wealdstone team for good, though I wish I hadn't, given how it happened. Dennis Byatt, who played centre half (and would go on to be Wealdstone's manager), went through a terrible tragedy – his young wife and baby both died in childbirth. I stepped in for Dennis and even ended up playing the F.A. Trophy semi-final against Enfield. But my first game was Frickley away on a freezing night – in fact, it was so cold that the Frickley fans built a big fire on the little hill behind the goal. The wind was howling and you couldn't see the goal because of all the smoke. We won 2–0, I think, though I'm not sure, given that we couldn't see anything.

Eventually, Dennis came back and I ended up on the bench for the F.A. Trophy final, and never got on against Boston. Wealdstone won that day, and won the league, becoming the first team to do the semi-pro non-league double. But I wanted more than a spot on the bench. What I got was a life-changing call from Dave Bassett and a taste of fame in northern Sweden.

There were two lads who played for Wealdstone – Nigel Johnson and Andy Divel – who spent part of the year playing in Scandinavia. When I heard about that, I wanted in. I still wasn't earning much at Wealdstone and I also wanted real playing time. I heard on the grapevine that the Swedish thing was partly brokered by none other than Dave Bassett, who'd watched me when I was an under-12. Back then, he'd told my manager, 'Keep me up to date on that kid', but as the years went by, he'd also gotten wind of some of my drink-fuelled shenanigans. So when I went to see Bassett to ask for his help in getting a pro gig in Scandinavia, his initial reaction was a big no thank you. But I told him, 'I'll get down on my hands and knees and I give you my word, nothing bad will happen.'

Apparently, Bassett called his contacts in Sweden and said, 'I've got this trialist, this young lad, and I need you to turn him into a man.' To me, a few days later he called and said, 'Right, you're going to Sweden, IFK Holmsund. Just stay out of trouble – no fighting, no aggro, nothing.'

And that's how, on 2 April 1986, I found myself 400 miles north-east of Stockholm in the town of Umea, on the Bay of Bothnia. Let's just say it wasn't exactly Miami Beach, but I loved it and I didn't get into a single scrap.

At the time, Holmsund were in the third division and I played one season as their centre half. I made the Swedish team of the week on multiple occasions, signed a bunch of autographs around town and I like to think that if I went back there they would raise a few tankards of Carnegie Porter to my time there (though mine's a Coke these days, thank you very much).

That season, Holmsund just so happened to play Djurgårdens IF in the Swedish Cup. Djurgårdens were a top-tier team – they even had Brian McDermott playing centre forward for them just a couple of years after he'd left Arsenal. Nevertheless, we beat Djurgårdens 4–2 – the equivalent of Accrington Stanley beating Manchester United. It was the lead item on all the news shows and in all the papers.

Holmsund were knocked out in the semi-final but by then I was heading back to England in any case – because Dave Bassett wanted me to sign for Wimbledon.

And I needed to be ready to meet Tanya Lamont again, though I couldn't have known it at the time.

Back then, one of the top teams in Sweden were Malmo FF and they were managed by none other than Roy Hodgson. He called Dave Bassett and told him that he wanted to sign me at the end of the Swedish season. Dave's response was to tell Roy that first he wanted to have a look at me, and then he'd decide.

So, I headed back to England and Wimbledon. They had just made it to the old First Division, not even a decade after they'd been elected to the Football League. When you think of how football has become so fossilized now, you can't imagine a little team making it from non-league to the Premiership, well, ever, right? I just don't think it could happen now, not with how much money is in the top of the game. But, just 30 years ago it was possible, and I was heading back to Wimbledon to see if I – and if they – could really make it in the top flight.

People talk about me, Dennis Wise, John Fashanu, all of them, being the Crazy Gang, but the original Crazy Gang was the Wally Downes team that had fought their way up the leagues. We just inherited the title.

But before I could make the Crazy Gang, I had to get in the team – and it was touch and go.

I was brought back for a month's trial. In fact, I'd still play for Wealdstone on Saturdays but train with Wimbledon during the week. During one practice match at Feltham, we found ourselves playing on a plastic pitch – horrible things, plastic pitches. (They don't play ice hockey on wood, or basketball on ice, so why does anyone play football on plastic? I just don't get it.) Anyway, I'm at centre back and the game is a disaster.

We were being watched by David Kemp, one of the Wimbledon coaches, and after the game he was talking to Derek French, one of the Wimbledon physios and a guy I'd known since I was a kid – in fact, he'd give me a ride to training every day, which meant that I got there two hours before everyone else, which was fine by me. But at the Feltham game, when the subject of Vinnie Jones comes up, Kemp said that it was clear I was not cut out to be a centre back at this level. Derek French did a head spin. 'Centre back?' French said. 'Vinnie Jones isn't a centre back. He's a centre midfielder, always has been.' Frenchy knew his football, and everyone knew Frenchy knew, thank god.

And then perhaps the most important stretch of my young career began.

A week or two later, on Tuesday 18 November 1986, there was another practice game, this time against Brentford. I was still a trialist, but now they'd put me in midfield and I managed to score twice in a 3–0 win. I also took the throw-ins and found I could hurl them as far as the penalty spot (I had no idea I had such a knack, but it was to serve me well). Luckily for me, the clubhouse was behind the field, and Dave Bassett, Dave Kemp and Frenchy the physio had been leaning out of the window, watching the game.

Wednesday was a day off; Thursday and Friday were jotted down for tactics, team selection, all that, ahead of the first team game at the weekend, which was against Nottingham Forest. At the time, Forest were a top team (they'd end the 1986–87 season eighth) – they had Neil Webb, Franz Carr, Cloughy's kid and Johnny Metgod, to name just a few. But Wimbledon had a player crisis: Stevie Galliers had been sent off in the previous game and Lawrie Sanchez was injured. Wally Downes was just coming back from injury, too. At the Thursday morning training session, if you got a blue bib, you were playing in the first team. Bassett threw Wally one . . . and then he threw me a blue one too. All the lads went, 'Fuck, mate, you're in!' Nottingham Forest away on Saturday.

At the end of the training session, I immediately went upstairs to Bassett's office. He said, 'Alright son, you're on 150 quid a week, 50 pound a goal, and 50 quid an appearance. I'm going to give you the rest of this year and next year. That's an 18-month contract to get into the first team and stay there.'

I was almost speechless, just about stammering out, 'OK.'

Then, when I managed to ask about a signing bonus, Bassett simply said, 'Go ahead and fuck off.' And that was my contract talks to join Wimbledon F.C. No agent, no photographers, no press conference, no Jim White going on about what a difference I'd make. Just a handshake, and a 'go ahead and fuck off'.

That night, I told my mate, Mark Robins, that I couldn't see him on Saturday because I'd be playing at Notts Forest. His dad, Basil Robins (god rest his soul), reportedly said, 'Vinnie needs help. He's a fucking lying little bastard and if he's blatantly fucking lying like that, well, to repeat, he needs some fucking help.'

On the Friday, I had to run to London to buy a suit. Bassett loaned me £150 to get it; it was my first suit (I've since bought a few more, bespoke). We travelled up to Nottingham that night, where the lads hazed me by sending a notorious woman called Amazing Grace to my room – somehow, I got her out before any harm was done, but not before she had sung a few rounds of 'If you're happy and you know it clap your hands' stark naked.

I suppose that's why they were known as the Crazy Gang.

I don't remember much about my first game, to be honest, which is a good thing, as I had a mare. We lost 3-2; I gave away a penalty after just 20 minutes, and in the most comical way you can imagine. And that wasn't even the worst part.

The penalty came about when the ball was crossed in from the left. I was tracking Neil Webb, or trying to – I'd been told he was future England captain material and my job was supposed to have been to mark him out of the game, but his movement and passing was just too good for me that day. After about 20 minutes we were one up, but then after a quick exchange of passes, Webb ran away from me in the box and swift-as-fuck Franz Carr whipped the ball in. I knew it was over me, and I wasn't having Webby bury it, so I just punched it away. I still remember all the Wimbledon lads going, 'Aww . . .' and turning away in resignation.

It was a long ride home. Back then, after away games we'd make a quick detour to drop Derek French off at his house and, because we were stopping anyway, we'd all pile into a pub called the Bell in Bedmond – right by where the M1 meets the M25 – before the bus made its way back into London to deposit the rest of the lads. That night in the Bell, I overheard one of Bassett's mates, Joe McGilliat, say, 'Harry! How can you put a fucking hod carrier up against Neil Webb for fuck's sake?'

I was devastated. I knew then it was over. Done. See you then. I'll let myself out. Just shy of 22 years old. One game for Wimbledon; punched the ball for a penalty; lost 3–2; Neil Webb for England; bosh.

But when the next week came around, injuries were still an issue. I learned much later that if Lawrie Sanchez had passed a fitness test, I wouldn't have played the next game and who knows if I'd ever have been able to get into the team ever again. But Lawrie failed his test and I was picked again. This time, it was at home against a little-known team called Manchester United.

At the time, United were struggling a bit; they'd sacked Ron Atkinson after a bad start to the season and they'd just hired a guy called Alex Ferguson from Aberdeen. The match on 29 November 1986 was only his fourth in charge (he went on to be their boss for 1,500 games!).

I remember that Saturday morning I had to go and buy some new boots – I can't remember what had happened to mine, but I had to run to a store called Peter Spivey's in Hemel Hempstead and buy some Nike boots (the store is still there). The boots were £27.50, I'll never forget. They weren't even leather.

It didn't matter though, as I scored the only goal of the game, with my head. We'd got a corner and, as Glyn Hodges swung the ball in, I leaped over Kevin Moran – *the* Kevin Moran, Irish international and first man to ever get sent off in a Cup Final – and hammered a header goalwards. Little Remi Moses was on the line and tried to clear it but I'd banged it so hard with my nut that I think it took a little bit of my scalp with it when it hit the roof of the net.

My celebration was ridiculous – I did a kind of Cockney knees-up thing then threw myself up against the railings (this was pre-Hillsborough) and tried to climb over. Some-one pulled me down, thank god. The ref lost his shit and ordered us all back to the half-way line sharpish and then I spent the rest of the match praying it would stay at 1–0. Bryan Robson even came on for them with about half an hour to go, but it was to no avail.

Wimbledon had beaten Manchester United 1–0 and I'd scored the only goal of the game in my second match ever in the First Division. A few months earlier I'd been playing for Wealdstone. Now, I'd just handed Alex Ferguson his second defeat as Man United manager. Clearly it wasn't going to work out for him there; everyone could tell.

At the end of the game I broke away from the lads as we made our way to the changing rooms and headed to the boardroom. I knew Joe McGilliat liked to hang out in there after games. I still had my kit on, my new boots, everything. But I didn't care. I charged into that board-room, went over to McGilliat and said, 'I'll bet you're glad I weren't fucking hod carrying today, weren't ya, you fucking bastard?'

That same weekend, a million miles from me (at least

emotionally), Tanya Terry was about half-way through her pregnancy with Kaley.

The rest of the season for me at Wimbledon was a mixed bag. After the United game we went to Stamford Bridge and won 4–0, and I'd scored again. Next game, Sheffield Wednesday came to Plough Lane and I scored *again* in a 3–0 win. After that the goals stopped, though, and I was about to get into my first real trouble on the pitch.

Arsenal came to Plough Lane and, before the game, curly-permed and mulleted Graham Rix had said that Wimbledon didn't deserve to play on the same pitch as the Gunners. (Let the record show that Arsenal ended that season fourth with seventy points and Wimbledon ended sixth, four points behind. So much for that theory, Mr Rix. And to show how much times have changed: Leicester City, who won the Premier League in 2016, and Manchester City, who won it in 2018 and 2019, were both relegated in 1987.)

Anyway, Rix's comments pissed me off, and I was determined to put him right. Maybe I did him with an elbow because my kit that day was sponsored by J&R Wrought Iron & Steel Construction; whatever it was, I clearly didn't heed the words of Dave Bassett in the matchday programme:

The game [against QPR] was marred by John Fashanu's dismissal, an event I hope will make him a wiser person . . . All players are aggressive, it's their nature, but John unfortunately gets more criticism than most . . . It doesn't help that he has a name that is a headline writer's dream. How many times have we seen

'Fash the Bash'? What we should do is change his name by deed poll to Arbuthnott-Jones then see what happens.

Weird that he'd pick Jones as a new name for Fash, because I was about to put my first mark on what would come to be a long list of moments that, when taken together, gave me the reputation for being a nutter.

We just thought, how dare you walk over us and think we're a piece of crap on your shoes? We took it personally; that was the Wimbledon way.

It was a tough school at that club back then. Legend has it that one poor player was initiated by his teammates by being tied to the top of a car and driven down the A3. You either grew a backbone or you dissolved. There were fights on the team bus – amongst ourselves. Alan Cork's car – a SEAT Toledo – was torched because Dave Bassett wouldn't give him a raise, so Cork was able to claim third party fire and theft.

But it was a family, of sorts, and right when I needed one. Bassett was the dad – or, more exactly, the chief warden. He would steam into you, but also be kind in other ways. Sam Hammam, the chairman, was a great and a kind character, too. Every Monday morning he'd sit with his solicitor in the transport café next to where we trained, waiting to find out what kind of trouble we'd gotten into that weekend and what he could do to fix it.

We weren't alone anymore; I had ten blokes behind me, and everyone else had ten blokes behind them. A few of us had had difficult upbringings. John Fashanu had been a Barnardo's kid; Dennis Wise had grown up without a lot of money. Wimbledon gave us a chance to prove ourselves, to be part of something.

So, for Graham Rix to suggest we weren't deserving of our place in the top flight ... well, Fash had given me a nickname – the Butcher – and I suppose I was taking that moniker a bit too much to heart. With Rix's slur running through my head, I threw an elbow his way early doors, but referee John Martin was having none of it and sent me off.

That was Saturday 17 April 1987. Bassett was so pissed off at me that, after I'd served my three-match ban, he refused to pick me for the final three games of the season, the first of which we won 1–0 at Old Trafford. It was a career-changing event for me.

And, though I didn't know it at the time, four days earlier, on the previous Tuesday 14 April 1987, Tanya Terry's life had changed forever, too.

5

A NEW HEART

There are so many odd connections in the world; I think all you have to do is be open to seeing them, really. My life with Tans taught me that there are coincidences everywhere you look that can't be explained, but that, if you're paying attention, can mean something important. Tans was certainly magically connected to these weird forces in the world – she often talked about her late grandad Tommy as though he was still alive, still present – and sometimes I felt I was just along for the ride.

Take a guy called Magdi Yacoub, for example. You may not have heard of him, but you really should have; he's far more important than any celebrity or politician or footballer. In fact, he was like a god in Tans' life because he *gave* her life, and so much more of it than she could ever have hoped.

Magdi Yacoub was born in 1935 in Egypt – his father was a surgeon and the Egyptian government moved them around a lot, so Magdi's early life was spent all over the country. It was a hard time to be going from place to place as a little kid, especially with war approaching. But Yacoub was a smart boy – he started school at three and by the time he was fifteen years old, he was deciding whether or not to be a doctor himself. His dad wanted him to do something else, but then something terrible happened, and it's one of those things that's a connection to a different time and place but which echoes down through our lives still.

Magdi's aunt – his dad's sister – sadly died in childbirth. Her heart had something relatively minor wrong with it, but the stress of the delivery and the fact that the simple fix for her problem wasn't available in Egypt at the time meant that they lost her. This tragedy finally convinced Magdi to be a heart surgeon, and all because a woman had heart trouble giving birth.

Fast forward decades, and Magdi is the main guy at a hospital called Harefield, in Hertfordshire. By the time Tans met him, he was an incredibly eminent man. He'd done the first heart and lung transplant on the planet, in 1983; and though I wish Tans had never had to meet Dr Yacoub, as she reverently called him, thank god he was there when she needed him.

I wish we had more of Tanya, more stuff to keep close, more things to hold, even more photos and mementos and videos to cherish. One thing we do have as a family, and which we feel so lucky to have found, is a diary she kept in the late 1980s about her heart transplant.

Kaley and I have been reading it in the months since we lost her and I'm going to share a lot of it here because it reveals just how brave she was, what she went through and how close we were to losing her then. She was so young; it's incredible to think that she faced her own mortality so early, and I think that's what ultimately made her what she was: someone who loved life so hard because it had almost been taken away.

As 1986 turned into 1987, Tans was approaching 21 years old, and she was pregnant for the first time. She'd been married for about a year to Steve and she was so excited to be having a child. She had been feeling a bit breathless in the later stages of her pregnancy, but doctors didn't pay much heed to it; it was probably just the baby squeezing out Tans' lungs a bit. But the baby was healthy and in the right position and that was all that seemed to matter.

In her diary she wrote:

From January to April of '87, I was so full of love and happiness. Pregnancy gives you natural contentment . . . I was round, glowing and loved everyone. I was always leaving little messages for my unborn child. I had more love in me for my living bump than I'd ever experienced before. Everything made me smile . . . Reading my diary of that time, I feel like I'm reading about someone else. I had such patience; I felt so calm and relaxed. I actually had everything. There was nothing I could have wanted except a secret yearning for a pretty little girl to spring into this world.

Tans went into labour on her actual twenty-first birthday if you can believe it: 14 April 1987. No snows that day; dry and warm. In fact, it was a perfect spring day.

Tans had started the day with breakfast in bed brought to her by Steve, and then had gone to see her nan, Ella, and her mum and dad. The weekend before she'd hung out with her posse of close friends – she always had so many close friends; that was Tans – and in her diary she lists them all: Joanne, Paula, Nicola and Julie. But by later on Tans' birthday, Joanne – who was herself engaged to Lee Sinnott, another Watford player – and Tanya's mum thought she was probably going into labour, so her mum took Tans to Watford General, the hospital literally next door to the Watford ground on Vicarage Road and the place where I'd been born too.

And that's when everything went wrong.

At the hospital, Tans was in a lot of pain, so they gave her an epidural. Tans always maintained that the epidural was what caused the problems (there are very rare cases where epidurals can cause heart issues). All it takes is for a nurse or doctor to get the insertion of the needle a little bit wrong and boom, major trouble. She said that after her epidural her body went tight and stretched and she felt her brain was going to pop out of her head. She could barely breathe, and this was before the baby had even started coming. That was her heart collapsing, but nobody realized. But she didn't want to panic because of the baby and, Tans being Tans, she pushed on through. By the next morning, Kaley was born:

The midwife told me I'd given birth to a Perfect Princess.
She was a browny-red with jet black hair; she seemed so

small . . . I loved her even more now that she was out in my arms.

But something was badly wrong:

My breathing became hard work. I asked for a wheelchair so I could be wheeled outside for some proper air – fresh and damp. I was put on the fire exit, all alone in the dark. I wish they had never bothered. I asked to be wheeled back in. I told a young nurse I was feeling a bit poorly and that my breathing felt strange . . . I turned my lamp on for attention and [the nurse] saw that my face was blue. She ran for the sister; there was a lot of panic . . . By this time my body was near frozen. I was wrapped in what I thought was giant tin foil . . . I knew I was desperately ill . . . I knew if I slept I would never wake up – I did not have the breath.

Tans was rushed to the ICU and a bunch of doctors pored over X-rays, but no one really knew what was what. Steve Terry, her mum and her friends all came to see her – but it was Joanne Southern's visit that freaked Tans out the most as Joanne couldn't help but cry, and Tans realized that Joanne must know something about her condition that she didn't. By this point, Steve is crying, Maureen is crying and a vicar has been to visit her.

When you know death is close it's a very lonely feeling; no one can do it for you. It is done only by you.

Fortunately – very fortunately – a heart surgeon was brought to see Tans and realized pretty quickly that something was very wrong. The decision was made to send Tans six miles down the road to Harefield Hospital; she didn't even know at that point that Harefield was a place where hearts got fixed.

By now, the doctors realized that she had suffered from something called cardiomyopathy. This means that her heart had swelled during pregnancy, but during the intense effort of labour, the same muscles that had swelled and been stressed by the pregnancy had collapsed. It had been a one-in-a-million chance that someone at the age of 21 should go through such a thing, but now she had just once chance to live: she needed a heart transplant. It was her only option, but even then, it was a really long shot.

Once at Harefield, things got really dire. On her first night, Tans was put in intensive care, which completely freaked her out. People were dying all around her on the ward, and she was terrified. Fortunately, a man called Dr Mitchell came to see her and calmed her down. He would become such an important part of our lives, that guy. He looked like a mad professor – he had crazy hair, like Christopher Lloyd playing the Dr Emmett Brown character in *Back to the Future* – but he was the kindest, and the best doctor you could ever imagine.

But first she had to wait – a full five weeks while the search went on for a new heart. Tans was moved out of the ICU to a regular ward to calm her down a bit. Dr Mitchell initially told Tans that it might be that she needed a pacemaker, but she was only 21 and a new mother and this devastated her. 'I might as well throw myself out of the window now,' she'd whispered to Mitchell.

Slowly, I got worse. I started to get thin and weak. I looked in the mirror one day and had a bad shock. I saw my eyes; it was awful. They seemed to be so far in my head. I knew I was dying.

Tans' diary is an incredible record of what she went through – all her fears and pain, but also evidence of the strength and love for her family, and mostly her love for Kaley.

The best way to explain how she made me feel is when I was breathless, she gave me breath. My wonder child.

Eventually, Dr Mitchell came to Tanya's bedside and told her she needed a heart transplant within the next two weeks – he was very straight with her and told her she would indeed die without it:

I was back on the monitors, right by the sister's room. My breathing became difficult again. From then on, all I remember is being moved back to ITU. How scary that was. Dr Mitchell had told me I needed a new heart in the next two weeks.
  My last memory of owning my old heart is laying with Steve, Mum and Dad. The hurt was just horrific. Watching

*my lovely mummy having to be taken out of the ITU. I
begged my dad to make sure my mum would be OK.*

*With Steve holding one hand and Dad holding the other,
very slowly my vision was going. Everything began to get
dark. It was very gradual. I told Steve very calmly I was
going now. It was definitely time to begin my journey to
heaven.*

*All the fear leaves you when it's time to die. All my
pain left me and for the first time in weeks I was actually
at peace. I had no strength left to fight for life. My heart
stopped there and then. [I was] knocking on heaven's door.*

Tans told Steve that she couldn't see; and suddenly the
room was filled with doctors and nurses rushing to save
her life.

I don't know how you live after this, I really don't. I do
believe it gave Tans a strong sense that life was so precious
and was to be filled with love and enjoyment. She had
always been a lovely person, but I think once this happened
to her, she got a strong look into what life is and what it
means to lose it. It also made her fearful, I think, of how
much a body can let you down.

That's just another reason why losing her has been so
terrible. She knew as much as anyone ever did how precious
life is. She never took it for granted, not one single day.

I don't think any of us should.

Tans was really funny, though, and I think that helped
her. Though she had been 'knocking on heaven's door' . . .

*. . . I can only presume God was not home, as I was sent
back again.*

*I was then put on a life support machine to keep me
alive while Dr Mitchell tried to find me a new heart. Mine
had completely stopped. Steve said the sound of the heart
monitor stopping will stay with him forever. He loved me
more than anything and he stood and watched me die. He
changed at that moment; that changed him completely. He
was never to be the same person again.*

I really don't know how two people who were so young
could go through so much. Don't forget, this all happened
in the two weeks after Tanya turned 21. Steve was four years
older, but he was still basically a nipper. They'd only gotten
married in June 1986; now, less than a year later, they'd just
had a baby and Tanya's heart had collapsed. I have nothing
but admiration for how Steve stayed with her throughout
that ordeal; it must have been terrifying. (He missed a lot of
Watford's games to be with Tanya – in fact, after Kaley was
born and Tanya's heart had collapsed, he only played one
more game all season – and he scored, with his foot! Pretty
good for a centre back with his mind elsewhere.)

Then, a miracle: a heart had been found for Tanya Terry.

For a heart to be found, sadly there had to be a tragedy
somewhere else – in this case, as far away as Germany. A
14-year-old boy had been involved in a car accident and
his family wanted him to be a donor. The heart had orig-
inally been designated for someone else – not Tans – but
the match had not been perfect. It was now mid-May.

Tanya had given birth five weeks earlier and was on life support; her need was the greatest of all in the transplant system, and the boy's heart fitted her needs perfectly.

But let's be clear: that's how close we came to losing her, way back in 1987. A chance accident on the autobahn 500 miles or so away? It doesn't bear thinking about – not for Tans, not for her family, not for the poor German family who lost their boy.

I think if you'd asked anyone around Tans – her mum, her dad, Shane, Steve, all her friends – they would have begged for any amount of extra time, given how incredibly close to death she came that spring. I suppose that Tans got 32 extra years was nothing short of a miracle – the record in the United States in 1987, the year she had her transplant, was a Stanford University School of Medicine heart recipient who had so far lived 18 years since his transplant. Though right now, a few months after losing her, even 32 years seems too short.

In her diary, Tans wrote that she was resigned to whatever is about to happen:

I knew nothing of all this. I thought I had gently left this beautiful, magic world and passed over to the other side to spend time with my precious grandad, Tommy. I believe that's why I had no fear; I knew Grandad, who I have always loved and respected, was waiting for me. I remember nothing of my time when I was dead. I just know the relief I felt . . . it was almost freedom to me for death to come at last. Peace is the best word that comes to mind.

The heart had been harvested in Germany, and now the agonizing wait for Tans' new heart to arrive at Harefield began. Tans' dad and Steve waited by the helicopter pad for hours, hoping to hear the whirr of the blades that would hopefully save her life. The last leg of the heart's journey had been by road, though, so before they knew it, wallop, Dr Yacoub and his team had started and completed the transplant. (In fact, helicopters would feature in many parts of our lives together, good and bad. But that's all to come.)

Yacoub found Lou and Steve and said, 'It's a good heart.'

Later, Tans would reflect on what it meant to get a new lease of life:

This was the only chance for me to live again, and be a daughter, a wife, and most important, a mother . . . I desperately wanted to be [that] for Kaley more than anything.

It was Monday 18 May 1987. The surgery had taken about eleven hours; eventually, Dr Yacoub emerged from the operating room to give Tans' family the good news that the transplant was complete and so far she was responding quite well. But she wasn't out of the woods:

The doctors were not sure if they had got the life support machine on in time. Once the heart stops it's only a matter of time before the oxygen stops getting to the brain. When this happens, if you manage to live again you can suffer brain damage. The doctors were quite sure this had happened to me.

Lou had gone home after the news about the possible brain damage and had stayed awake all night, terrified and devastated. This darling daughter of his, to whom he'd always been so close; the girl he'd held in his arms when she was born between a football match and the boxing, the proudest man in the world; the girl he'd waved off to Lea Farm School, trying to swallow the great lump in his throat; the 12-year-old he'd brought Persephone home to as a surprise for her birthday; the woman he'd given away to Steve Terry . . . after everything they'd all been through, this was the cruellest blow. To have faced losing her, only to have this news about her brain – her brilliant, quirky, love-filled brain – follow on the heels of the baby and the transplant, well, it seemed to everyone like the universe's worst ever joke.

But then something magical happened, yet again. Lou and Steve and Maureen were allowed into the ante room in the ICU the next morning for a second and they all stood looking at Tans, devastated that she might have suffered a terrible brain injury. They couldn't see her face, so couldn't tell if she was OK or not.

And it was at that moment that a little hand appeared from under the sheet and waved. Their daughter, Steve's wife, Tanya Terry, had just waved at them – her dad and her mum knew there and then that she was fine, because you know your child more than you know anything in the world and they could just feel it.

Their little girl was going to be OK.

It was time for Tanya to begin her life all over again.

She was in intensive care and out of it for the rest of the week, until Friday.

Friday morning, 22nd May, Shane's birthday, was the first day of my new life. I had been asleep since leaving my life on Monday afternoon.

But it was still a really hard thing to understand for such a young woman:

The real pain and horror hit me – I had had a heart transplant. The ache around my chest and lungs was horrific and I was totally numb with shock . . . I asked for a mirror. The moment Mum had dreaded . . . In my whole life, I had never seen anything so ugly. The scar down my chest was disgusting. I had so many stitches . . . I knew at that moment my life would never be the same again. I thought there could be nothing worse than that until I lifted the mirror to my . . . face. I looked like a bloated hamster, and I was yellow. I was devastated . . . I don't think I even asked after my darling Kaley that day. All I wished was that my family had been brave enough to ask the doctors to turn the life support machine off so I could have died with beauty and dignity.

Eventually, Tans started to feel a bit more hopeful:

After a couple of days, I learned to walk, very slowly. I started to wash myself and gradually became a little independent, which made me a tiny bit happier.

Looking back, though, I was confused, shocked and very depressed. I had always been a happy person; I had never suffered from depression, so I did not understand this emotion. I believe I was mentally unstable too, and that probably lasted 18 months . . . at least.

Failure was the feeling I could not cope with, and being ill and relying on everyone to do everything for me made me feel like I had failed . . . How can a woman not have a baby easily? What did I do wrong? Why did my healthy heart collapse? Why why why, that's all I ever asked. I drove myself mad wondering, doubting myself, doubting Steve, doubting God, the doctors, nurses, my family, my friends, just doubting everything. Again [I was] wishing I could have peacefully died.

The depression continued to affect her marriage, though, and her role as a new mum:

Every day when I watched Steve walk in, I doubted my love for him; I think he felt the same. He had had six weeks preparing for my death and here I was alive. He was shocked at me surviving and he knew I had become totally dependent on him.

I was [also] frightened at the thought of being a mummy, suddenly. Before all this I was confident I would be a perfect young mum. Now I felt like a child again who needed looking after; I was now frightened of the thought of looking after a baby all by myself.

As ever, Kaley saved the day:

The day my love Kaley was brought to me all my sadness left me. I remembered how she made me feel. All my proudness came back, all my love filled my body again.

One day, Maureen was pacing her living room, worried sick about her daughter. It was a terrible time for everyone, but imagine a mother having to watch her only daughter fight for her life, and also be unable to fully enjoy her first grandchild, given the circumstances. Maureen describes it as the worst moments of her life . . . and right in the middle of that toughest of days, the phone rang. She was afraid it was the hospital; how wrong she was.

'Hello, Maur,' said a voice. 'It's Elt, here.'

This rang no bells.

'Who is it?' Maureen said, exasperated.

'Elt,' said the voice.

Maureen had no idea. She was on the verge of just putting the phone down.

'No, I heard that,' said Maureen. 'But who is it, who is it?'

'It's Elt, Elt, Elton John.'

There was a pause, and then Maureen said, 'Jesus Mary and Joseph!'

God bless his heart, he was calling to see whether or not to send Tans real or fake flowers (Tans' room had to be kept sterile, of course, so fake it was). The Rocketman even went to see Tans in hospital, sitting on the end of her bed and chatting with her. That was during the time Elton was married to Renate Blauel and Renate used to call Tans now and then. (Once she was out of hospital, Tans went to a party Elton threw in Chorleywood; she even called Dr Mitchell beforehand to see if she was allowed to have a glass of champagne. She was.) And for the rest of her life, Elton has always remembered to ask after her whenever I've seen him; what a great guy.

And beyond Kaley and Steve and her family and friends like Elton John, there was one other person who helped Tans more than I think he ever knew:

My favourite, Dr Mitchell, would come by from time to time . . . He was always so honest with me and frank, but from the moment I met him there was always a home in my heart for him; there still is. He is the cleverest man I ever met. Even now when I see him I need him to reassure me that he will never leave Harefield Hospital. I always think the day he leaves is the day I will die. I need him.

After Tans died, I spoke to Dr Andrew Mitchell to thank him for everything and to tell him what Tans had thought of him. I said, 'She spoke so highly of you – you were her knight in shining armour.' He was in shock when I told him that; that's how great and selfless that guy is. He's a true, real, lifesaver and he had no idea.

And then it was Monday 1 June 1987 – exactly two weeks after Tans' heart transplant:

Finally, the day came. I heard the words, 'Tanya, would

you like to go home?' What a feeling. If I could still do back flips, I would have done a hundred. The drive was wonderful; the sun, the green grass, the smell of summer, the horses, sheep and cows in the fields, the blue sky, the white clouds. My jaw ached from smiling by the time I got home to Mum's.

The best thing in life must be your Mum's house, the house you spent your whole childhood [in], the happiest time. [My childhood was] a special, special time, and although I had gone, it was in my own memory box. I cried and cried from happiness. I never thought I'd see Gaddesden Crescent again, my favourite place in the whole world. My roots.

Waiting for her, in a crib, was her new baby.

Kaley laying in her crib gave me a warm glow. Her beauty kept shocking me. Her skin was like silk.

By this time, she was quite fair. She was ten weeks old. My very own perfect daughter.

But still the depression stalked her. Maureen remembers that she was hanging the washing one day while Tanya went to have a bath. Glancing in the mirror, Tanya had been horrified at what she'd seen. Maureen heard her crying and screaming. Rushing up to her, Tanya tearfully confessed she felt like she resembled an ape, as the steroids had caused dark black hair to grow on her body.

All these changes made Tans very anxious:

Sometimes I would feel strangely homesick for Harefield. Although I did not want to spend my life in hospital, I knew I was safer there. I was so afraid, suddenly, of dying; it began to take over my every thought. One moment I would be fine and laughing and chatting – next thing, I would be howling and screaming out of control. The fear feeling did not leave me for at least 18 months.

There were dangerous physical issues, too.

Tans had only been home for a few days when she suffered a fit caused by the drugs she had to take. She was rushed back to hospital, where she had to stay for a few days; she was vomiting and in a lot of pain. She suffered a punctured lung and had to have it drained for 48 hours. But she finally made it home for good, and then to her friends Joanne and Lee Sinnott's wedding, where she was a bridesmaid. But that was to be as happy as she got for a while:

Joanne's wedding day was to be my last happy day for a very long time. Kaley made me happy, Steve too, but I was so unhappy with myself, the way I felt and looked. My hair and my eyebrows started to change colour. I completely lost my confidence and would find myself crying for hours and not knowing why.

For two years, Tans covered herself up to her chin, she was so embarrassed by that scar running down her chest. She told the *Sun*:

I've got photographs that I can't even look at because I can't
believe it's me. I was covered up for two and a half years.
I wouldn't leave the house unless I was dressed up to my
chin. I was devastated for two years, but one day I thought,
'What am I doing? This is part of me now.'

There was some comfort, too, in the form of 'visits' from
grandad Tommy. Tans was adamant he'd come to her and
sit on the end of her bed; he was always in his uniform and
his presence calmed her. They had always been so close, it's
not surprising to me that she felt he was with her at such a
difficult time.

Now, I feel Tans' presence, too. Recently I came home
from a day at the golf course and I was eating a meal Kaley
had made. It tasted just like how her mum made it and it
conjured up Tans for me so strongly that I felt she was there,
in that room, sitting with me as she always did, asking me
about who I'd played with and how I'd played and what
everyone had said and what the weather had been like
and whether or not I'd had a good time ... and I couldn't
look over to the couch where Tans used to sit, because even
though I could feel her presence that night and hear her
beautiful voice and sense her everywhere – how she looked
and sounded and smelled, and the huge smile she had,
lighting up for all of us, all the time – if I turned my head
and looked to my right, to that couch where once she'd
sat, Tans wasn't actually going to be sitting there anymore,
and not seeing her there would have ruined me. So I kept
looking straight ahead, blankly staring at the TV, eating the

meal Kaley had made and missing my Tans more than it's possible to write or think or say.

Late that summer of 1987, with her new heart beating just fine inside her and her love for Kaley deepening with every minute, Tans had to face another jolt: the new football season had arrived and Steve, who'd missed a bunch of games when Tans had been so sick, had to head off to Sweden for pre-season training.

Tans writes that she could never have imagined life without Steve, and he wanted her life to get back to something like normal, so he told her to go out with all her mates and have a good time. But when Tans finally got around to having a night out, with Maureen on babysitting duty, it was so painful, despite her best efforts:

I felt the whole world was looking at me and talking about me. I could not stand it. I shook all night and felt like I was on show.

That night, I realized how much my life and myself had changed. I was no longer the fun-loving, carefree girl in the crowd. I was suddenly Tanya Terry, the Heart Transplant Survivor.

From then on, Tanya had a regimen of drugs she had to take, drugs that she was still taking right up to the end . . . or almost the end. One of the key drugs was cyclosporin, which works to shut down the part of the immune system responsible for rejecting foreign tissue, but is also a drug that can increase the chance of certain cancers. We'd come to see those side effects all too clearly as the years passed.

There were times, too, in the first years after the transplant, where Tans swallowed her tongue a few times – Steve would have to put his hand down her throat to save her. She would have seizures too, because they were still going through a kind of trial and error with some of her medications. It must have been a really hard time for everyone.

We'd learn later that what kept her heart going was probably what led to all her health issues at the end. It seems so unfair; but then, everything seems unfair now, without her.

6

PRINCESS DI AND STEVE McMAHON AND PRINCESS DI AGAIN

As Steve Terry went off to my old stomping ground of Sweden to do his pre-season training, Wimbledon's pre-season training for the 1987–88 season didn't get off to the best of starts – we'd lost our leader. Dave Bassett had left Wimbledon in the summer of 1987 to go to manage Watford and I was pretty sure I'd follow him. For a start, it was my club, and second, I'd have followed Bassett anywhere.

After Bassett moved to Watford, I went to meet him and Elton John at Vicarage Road during a reserve game. We talked about a possible move and, as the conversation wound down, Elton said, 'Where are you going now?' And I said, 'Up the pub, the Bell, to have a pint.'

'You don't mind if I come up and have a beer on the way, do you?' he said.

Fifteen minutes later, we all arrived at the Bell in Bedmond; me in my car with Bassett and Elton in his Rolls

Royce Silver Spur with driver. The locals couldn't believe their eyes. We had a few beers and then all of a sudden Elton just said, 'Right, I'm off then. We'll get the deal done. I'll speak to Sam in the morning.'

But Sam Hammam was having none of it, so I stayed.

In came Bobby Gould, a very different kind of fella to Bassett. To help him with the training, Gould hired Don Howe, who we all loved – what a brilliant tactician he was.

But first, Gould had to navigate the ways of Wimbledon chairman Sam Hammam.

Gould wanted to buy Terry Gibson from Manchester United to improve our defence. The price was £250,000, which Hammam was happy to pay, as long as Gould ate 12 sheep testicles (Hammam also had it written in our contracts that if we ever lost 4–0 we had to attend the opera).

New players came in, and we tested them hard to see if they had what it took to be a part of the Crazy Gang. John Scales hated it; Terry Phelan later said that for the first six months at Wimbledon, he had no dreams. 'I used to sit in the bedroom and say my career is gone; where do I go from here?' Phelan said. Players were locked in the boot of a car, dragged around in the snow, forced to not eat for two whole days. It wouldn't be tolerated now, but then, it was how we did things.

And it started to work, at least in the F.A. Cup. We battered West Brom in the third round, 4–1 at home; then Mansfield Town 2–1 away in round four. In the fifth round we beat Newcastle United in the north-east, 3–1, and then the tie that had all of us, but especially me, wincing: at home to Dave Bassett's Watford (and Watford had Steve Terry at centre back too). We let in a bad goal by their Malcolm Allen and then our centre back, Brian Gayle, punched Allen in the throat and got sent off. Somehow, we turned it around to win 2–1, though poor Gayley never played for the rest of the cup run, which I always thought was a terrible thing to do to him.

We went a goal down to Luton Town in the semi-final but came back again to win 2–1. Now we were headed to Wembley to face mighty Liverpool in the F.A. Cup Final. (Months earlier, and again affronted by the egos of the bigger clubs, I'd written 'Bollocks' on a piece of tape and stuck it across that poxy sign in the Liverpool tunnel, thereby changing 'This is Anfield' to 'This is Bollocks'. We were barred from the players' lounge for that, I'm proud to say.)

So just three years after I'd watched Watford head to Wembley, and told myself I'd be there one day, that day had arrived; I couldn't believe it. Sam Hammam gave an interview which summed up how we all felt: 'If Wimbledon can do it, anyone can do it.'

The build-up to the game had all been about how we didn't deserve to be there and that we were going to get hammered. The prospect of such a humiliation drove us on. One intro to the game called Liverpool 'the greatest post-war club we've seen'. Their team was filled with stars, not least of whom was a Watford old boy, and former neighbour to Tans, John Barnes. He was no longer living with Annie Nicell on Gaddesden Crescent, and he'd lost one Cup Final with Watford (the one in which Tans had told Barnes' wife that she recognized me from the bus). Surely, he wouldn't lose another, not with this Liverpool team around him.

But Don Howe had done a brilliant thing. He'd said, 'To stay in this level, you need the quickest back four in the country. They might not be able to play football, they might not be able to pass water, but they need to be the quickest in order to get back and tackle.' And that's what Gould put together: he got Keith Curle, who ended up a good player; John Scales and Terry Phelan, who was probably one of the quickest lads I played with over 60 yards – in fact, he was always having hamstring problems because he was so fast. There was Eric Young, quick as fuck; Andy Thorn over 60 yards was very speedy and Clive Goodyear didn't look it, but he was no slouch over 100 metres either. So we had the quickest back four in the league and it would stand us in great stead in the heat of the Cup Final.

On the field before the game I couldn't get the smile off my face. I was natty in a grey suit and blue and cream mottled tie, but as a team we were scared. And we fed off that fear. In the tunnel we were shouting 'In the hole!' – a reference to an unfortunate moment previously when I'd promised Kenny Dalglish that if he fouled me again, I'd rip his head off and shit in the hole.

But before we could get at Liverpool, we had to line up and meet Princess Di. Imagine me, a lad who two years before was playing for Wealdstone, now on the famous Wembley turf shaking the hand of the most famous woman in the world.

I wonder if Tans was watching that day. I wish I could

ask her. I know her dad was, because he's told me. But no one can remember if she watched. She was never much of a football watcher. But according to Kaley, she sure liked the hot dogs.

Fourteen minutes into the final I smashed Steve McMahon, just to prove that we didn't give a shit. That tackle was planned weeks earlier; we'd noticed that McMahon would show for a ball in from the full back, turn and play it the opposite way. Well, I was waiting for him.

It was a crunching tackle, let's say. On the way down, he elbowed me and split the skin under my eye – fair play to him for that. Referee Brian Hill just pointed for the free kick and on we went. These days I'd be sent off for a leveller like that, no question. Fash said the tackle 'started at [McMahon's] neck and ended at his ankle', which seems about right.

On 37 minutes, Dennis Wise whipped in a great free kick, and Lawrie Sanchez glanced a header past Bruce Grobbelaar; 1–0 to the Crazy Gang. After an hour, John Aldridge went down in the box – penalty. It was clearly a great tackle by Clive Goodyear. Afterwards, even Aldridge, in all fairness, said it wasn't a penalty. When pens like that are given, you do wonder if the fix is in; would the powers that be really let a team like Wimbledon beat a team like Liverpool?

But just because the ref gave them a dodgy pen, doesn't mean you automatically score them . . . and it's sometimes made harder when your opponent keeps yelling that you're going to miss it, as we all did to John Aldridge. Aldridge stepped up and fired it to Dave Beasant's left, but Dave flung himself and turned it around the post. It was the eleventh penalty Aldridge had taken that season and the first he'd missed; it was also the first penalty ever saved in an F.A. Cup Final.

We were going to do it; we were really going to do it.

At the final whistle, my socks around my ankles, I put my arms up in the air and almost accidentally hugged the ref. Then I went running off to celebrate; I didn't know where. On the telly, John Motson was saying that the Crazy Gang had beaten the Culture Club. He also said, 'Her Royal Highness applauds one of the great cup shocks of all time. It's a weird and wonderful world if you come from Wimbledon. The background from which these players have come has made the moment all the more satisfying. They couldn't have dreamed it, one or two of them, bearing in mind where they were two or three years ago.'

He got that right, did Motters.

But, me being me, there was still controversy to create. I felt like it was my day; the press, who'd counted us out, couldn't take my medal away from me. To most people, we were scum, we were nothing, and they would see our victory as a disaster in football history. And those feelings of anger at how we'd been written off just came out of me that afternoon. And in my fervour to point out that we'd had the balls to win, I banged my gonads into Bobby Gould's face (he was kneeling on the Wembley turf and was wearing the actual F.A. Cup trophy on his head at the time). Gould wasn't happy about it, but I'd made my point – it took stones to do what we'd done.

The celebrations never seemed to end; I even went to the Bell in Bedmond to see my mates. But eventually I headed home, to a new house I'd just bought in Hemel Hempstead: 5 Hunter's Oak.

I thought this was my life, started for real. I'd won the cup, I was Jack the Lad, I was in magazines and all the back pages. Little did I know that my real life was yet to start, right there along Hunter's Oak.

7

GEORGE THE RABBIT

I have had my new heart for four years today. I do not feel very happy though as now it's broken.

– from Tanya's diary, 18 May, 1991

The rest of my life started thanks to George.

George is a rabbit. (Or was. He had an unhappy end, but we'll come to that.)

Things went south at Wimbledon pretty quickly after the Cup Final win. The season following it was disastrous for me. It had started badly: on a pre-season tour of the Isle of Wight, I'd gotten into it with a defender called Dave Woodhouse who was playing for what amounted to a village team. Bobby Gould, the manager who'd taken us to the island for some obscure reason, had been livid that I'd gotten sent off and suspended me from the team, meaning I missed the Charity Shield (he might have still been pissed about the moment after the Cup Final when I'd shaken my stuff at him – who knows?).

After that, things only got worse – that season I was

blamed for ending Gary Stevens' career with a tackle, but if you watch the video it's clear I got the ball (I'd also gone right through my mate John Fashanu, who was tussling with Stevens, so there was no intent to hurt anyone – why would I try to injure my own teammate?)

Then, a few months later, in a game against Everton, I caught Graeme Sharp with a late one on the top of his boot and, in the subsequent melee, Kevin Ratcliffe did his best Meryl Streep impression by pretending I'd headbutted him – honestly, if I had, he wouldn't have gone down in stages. (I actually think they had to add some extra time at the end of the game to make up for how long it took him to swan dive to the turf. I've worked with some great actors in Hollywood, but Ratcliffe that day? 'And the award goes to . . .') Of course, it being me, I got sent off again and it was clear that Bobby Gould and his assistant, Don Howe, were getting to the end of their tether. My reputation was that I was a nutter and that I couldn't play football, but do you really think a guy who won the F.A. Cup wasn't any good? Yes, I was tough, and some of my tackles were as sharp as cheddar, but I never set out to hurt anyone. And I could play a bit; my first touch was solid, I could pass and shoot, I was good in the air, I scored goals and I was a leader.

None of it mattered. By the end of the 1988–89 season, Leeds United were interested in me and when Sam Hammam makes up his mind, he makes it up quickly. And so I was off to Elland Road.

Off the field, things were great. I was now a fully-fledged star; I had a nice little three-bedroom house on Hunter's

Oak and now I had a big move to Leeds United. I rented out the Hunter's Oak house and moved north.

I did a year at Elland Road, then I went to Sheffield United – which was a disaster on the field, though off it I became a father to a little boy called Aaron (me and his mum didn't last) – and then I moved back south to sign for Chelsea. I got rid of the renters and moved back into my house on Hunter's Oak.

At the time there was a great lad playing for Chelsea called Joe Allon. Joe was from Newcastle – he was one of Gazza's mates and he was hilarious. But back then, even though he'd been transferred from Hartlepool to Chelsea (imagine that happening now!), when he came south, he was living above a pub in Beaconsfield, of all places. We hit it off brilliantly, and as he was in a fix with his digs, I had him move in with me at number five. (Of course, given what people thought at the time, Joe's subsequent lack of success at Chelsea, where he only played 14 times and scored twice, was blamed on yours truly. The soccer rag *When Saturday Comes* wrote, 'Rumours in Hartlepool suggested Joe and his flatmate, Vinnie Jones, had hooked up with an old mate from Newcastle days called Paul Gascoigne and that lager-fuelled mayhem had been unleashed on west London.' Which was bollocks, by the way. But it shows that my reputation wasn't doing me any favours.)

I wasn't done with trying to fill the house, either. Yet another friend, Dell, had been kicked out by his missus (Maureen – she later became my housekeeper in Watford of all things). So sure enough, Dell moves in, too. So now we have a proper bachelor pad. We're living the life. Or, we think we are.

I was still single, and I could never imagine it any other way. Maybe I still held a flame for Tanya Lamont who was now Tanya Terry – who knows? Either way, I wasn't about to settle down; I was playing for Chelsea in the top flight, I had a F.A. Cup winner's medal and I was finally on some good money. Deep down did I wonder what it would be like to have a real relationship? Probably. But in any case, lightning, in the form of a fucking rabbit, was about to strike.

One day after training, Joe and I were sitting at home when we heard laughing from outside. Joe went to the window to report what was happening.

'Oh my god,' Joe said, 'there's them girls from next door again.'

I said, 'What do you mean, next door?'

'There's three girls that live next door – didn't you know? One of them has a kid . . .'

This was obviously excellent news for three single men, two of whom played for Chelsea. I joined Joe at the window just in time to see a woman in cut-off jeans with beautiful long hair glide by like a supermodel on roller skates. She had a little girl with her.

It was the most beautiful sight you can imagine. They looked so happy, rolling up and down Hunter's Oak in the late afternoon light. I kept trying to get a glimpse of the woman, but the sun was low and I couldn't make out her face. Joe and I were transfixed with these two, though –

they looked so angelic, doing pirouettes, holding hands and screeching with laughter.

And then the woman turned towards 5 Hunter's Oak and with the sun behind the houses at last, I could finally catch a glimpse of her face.

'Oh my god, Joe,' I said.

'What, mate?'

'It's Tanya.'

'Tanya?'

I'd last seen Tanya during the Suzuki debacle when she was 17; since then, she'd clearly turned into a woman. I'd read in the local paper about her heart transplant – it had been big news in Watford – and had been sorry to hear what she'd been through. Now, though, she must've been 24 or 25, and she still had those big, beautiful eyebrows, though her hair was even thicker than before. If she was the other side of the M1 from me back when we were teenagers, now she was five fucking M1s away from me; in fact, we weren't even in the same country.

'Yes, mate,' I said to Joe. 'It's Tanya. I knew her when she was Tanya Lamont, from years ago. She's married to Steve Terry now. She had a heart transplant. What the fuck is she doing on Hunter's Oak with her kid?'

Joe said, 'I spoke to her yesterday.'

'What?'

'She's married to Steve Terry.'

'I know, mate, I just told *you* that.'

'Oh, right,' said Joe.

'Well, what you fucking talking to her for?' I said. I didn't need Joe Allon – or anyone – talking to Tanya. Not. At. All.

'Her rabbit got out,' Joe said. 'Her little daughter's rabbit got out of the thing. I caught it and took it back to the whatchamacallit?'

'The cage, mate. It's called a cage. Maybe a hutch.'

'Right,' Joe said. 'The fucking thing was running around the street. It had a taste of freedom. Well, I say running. It was actually hopping. Anyway, I distracted it, corralled it, and took it back.'

This could only mean one thing. I had bought a house on a street in Hemel Hempstead, and now Tanya and Steve Terry and their kid lived next door. I'm not much of a mathematician, but I'd like someone to do the odds on that happening and I'd still never take that bet. As Rick says in *Casablanca*, 'Of all the gin joints in all the towns in all the world, she walks into mine.'

We both watched in awe as the light faded and Tanya and her daughter roller skated up and down our street.

'I am a fucking hero, mate,' Joe said, referring, I think, to the rabbit.

A few days later, I happened to glance out of my bedroom window when who should I see but Steve Terry pulling up next door. A few minutes later, I noticed that he was putting the little girl in a car seat and then he drove away.

You didn't need to be Inspector Clouseau to work out what was going on: Tanya and Steve must have split up. Later that day I asked Joe what he knew. He told me that Tans was living with a couple of other young women next door. One of them was Joanne Southern, who had gone to my school, Langleybury, and had been the one crying at Tans' bedside when her heart had collapsed. Joanne had had a massive crush on me back then, apparently; she used to sit there all dinnertime watching me play football in the playground.

Well, now she was living next door with Tanya and Steve Terry had signed for Northampton Town. He was living there full time and had a girlfriend. It turned out that he and Tanya had bought the house next door to me a few months after I'd moved in but things hadn't worked out. They'd tried to stay together for the kid's sake, but eventually they'd split up. So now Tanya was living with her daughter, Joanne and another girl, and right next door it was me, Joe Allon and Dell. Some days I'd see Tanya's little girl, Kaley, sitting on my wall, dangling her legs. Little did I know that Kaley, even back then a Man United fan if you can believe such a thing, was singing a little ditty about Chelsea players like me. She likes to remind me of this whenever she gets the chance:

Chelsea are rubbish
We know what to do
Flush all the players
Down the loo
Woo.

Quite the poet, our Kaley.

Now, not to give any credence to what *When Saturday Comes* thought of my living arrangements, but our house was, in all honesty, a bit of a carnage, shall we say? There were girls coming and going, lads coming and going – it was party time. We certainly did our fair share contributing to the bottom line of local watering holes, let's say that.

For her part, Tans had realized I was next door and was dubious to say the least. She later told the *Sun*:

When I first saw him again, he was a skinhead with a diamond ear stud, and I was so shocked. I thought, 'Oh god, he's a thug.' I used to read things about him and think, 'how irritating'. I kept telling myself I hated him but every time I saw him my insides turned over. I was always looking for him.

One evening we were all in the pub and I was trying to have a good time, but something wouldn't leave me alone – my brain kept fixating on something and I couldn't quite put my finger on it. But everyone started to notice that I wasn't really there, and let me be clear: when I'm there, I'm there full on and then some. But not that night, not at all. At about 9 p.m. I gave up and left; I felt like my clothes didn't fit, or something, or I'd got a pebble in my shoe. Maybe it was the fly, leather New York Yankees hat I was wearing (in Hemel Hempstead); who knows.

For a while, whenever I arrived back at 5 Hunter's Oak, I'd have the music up really loud in case it made Tans come out. I didn't mind if she was annoyed, I just wanted to see her.

And then on the way home from the pub my brain cleared and I realized I was thinking exactly one thing: how do I get to actually talk to her, rather than just annoy her with The Clash or Madness? Back at Hunter's Oak, I snuck up to Tanya's front window and looked in – she was sitting in an armchair and there was a lad sitting on the couch. My heart sank; I remember saying out loud, 'Oh, fucking hell. Whatever.'

There was nothing to be done, so I went to bed, my heart heavy. It was a warm night, so I left the windows open to let a nice breeze in . . . who am I kidding? I wanted to hear if the lad would leave or something. Actually, I don't really know what I was thinking; my mind was still racing with that maddening thought: how do I get to talk to her? I knew she was several M1s beyond me, but I was right back at Sun Sports and Gaddesden Crescent, thinking about how to talk to her.

I was starting to doze off when I heard voices . . .

'Yeah. OK then. Thanks a lot. Bye bye.' Wallop – I'm at the window. The lad was in his car by this point and I watched as he drove off.

It was my chance. I put my clothes back on – not the leather Yankees hat, mind – and I rushed downstairs. Trying to be cool, I slowed down a bit and walked up to her door.

Vincent Jones had a plan.

Knock knock. She answers. 'Oh my god, Vincent,' Tans said. 'Vincent Jones.'

So far so good. And then I put my plan into action.

'I just found your rabbit running around in the alley,' I said, 'and I've just taken it around to the garden and put it back in its hutch.'

It's not just Joe Allon who gets to be a hero.

'Really?' Tanya said.

'Yes,' I said. 'I was worried it was going to get run over or something. Can't be having that.'

'That's funny,' Tanya said, pointedly *not* inviting me in.

'Oh?' I said, getting the feeling the plan wasn't as watertight as I'd hoped.

'Yes,' said Tanya. 'You see, we put a padlock on the door of the hutch a few days ago.'

Now, it's not like I wanted the ground to open up or anything, but I wouldn't have minded a quick tornado to spin down the street, or an earthquake maybe. Anything to take our minds off the fact that I'd just told one hell of a porker.

But I didn't need an earthquake, because Kaley decided to get involved, even though she was only little. Suddenly, from upstairs, we could hear her calling out – she was probably three or four at the time.

Tanya said, 'Can you wait a minute? My daughter's crying.' But still she didn't invite me in. Instead, she kind of pushed the door to and ran upstairs. I was thinking, 'So we met when we were 12 years old. We had the Suzuki incident at 18. Now we live next door to each other. She's single. I'm single. I'm letting myself in.'

And that's what I did. I stepped into that house, shut the door behind me and started my new life, right there and then.

The first thing I did in that new life was put the kettle on and find a packet of custard creams.

By the time the kettle was about to start whistling, Tanya was coming back downstairs. Naturally enough, she went to the front door, thinking I was still on the step. Not seeing me there, she came into the kitchen to find me with half a custard cream in my gob.

Tanya wasn't impressed.

'What's going on?' she said.

'Well,' I said, 'you took so long I thought I'd better make a cup of tea.' We can thank the after-effects of the beers I'd had earlier in the evening for that line. I was filled with a kind of stupid courage.

'You're so cheeky,' she said, still unimpressed.

And then we sat down with our cups of tea and our biscuits and we talked until five in the morning.

I would have kept talking past five, but I had to get to training.

It had been the most incredible night of my life. We'd shared everything – literally everything we could think of to share. I told her my whole life story up to now — Mum and Dad splitting up, running from couch to couch, blowing my chances at Watford, heading to Sweden, coming back to England to play in my own Cup Final, then Leeds, Sheffield and the son I had, and Chelsea, and now this: the two of us talking all night.

She told me about Steve, and Kaley, and the heart transplant, and the break-up. There were tears, and we laughed a lot too, but mostly we just talked and talked and talked until I had to leave to go to Chelsea.

As I got up to go, I went to give her a kiss on the cheek.

'What?' she said, pushing me away. 'Certainly not.'

I tried something else: 'Here's my number,' I said.

'I don't need your number,' Tans said, 'because I will never call you. I've never rang a man in my life.'

(As for George . . . I found out years later he froze to death in the garden. He couldn't come in the house because Tans had to be extra careful about infections. Thanks anyway, George.)

That day at the training session, I ran faster than I ever had before, and I was known for winning every training race anyway. But I could have run through a brick wall that morning. Where my life had been 90 per cent or sometimes even 100 per cent, now it was a million per cent.

And it wasn't just me, apparently. In a diary entry dated July 1992, Tanya wrote:

Today I fell in love with someone I hardly know,
and I let myself imagine he could love me so.
I forgot how beautiful butterflies in my tummy felt.
I never dreamt – Vincent Jones you've been gone so long –
would be my awakening.
I love it.

Some months later, Tanya told me that she'd had a quick nap after I'd left, gotten Kaley up and off to school and then had called her mum.

'Mum,' she said, breathless. 'I've got to come see you. What time's your lunch?'

When Tans arrived, and before they'd even properly sat down, her mum said, 'What's his name?' Her mum knew straight away, probably because, as Tans later put it, 'I was lit up like a Christmas tree.'

'It's Vincent Jones,' Tans said. 'We've been up all night talking.'

But Tans was a tough nut to crack.

A few days later I asked Tans if she might be going to the local golf club that weekend; I knew her dad sometimes went. She said she was indeed going, though that had been a fib; she apparently called all her friends to come with her. I had my dad and my uncles with me, and we all ended up in my back yard. I thought it was going OK, but Tans announced she had to leave, so I had to move fast.

'Dad, go home,' I said.

It wasn't nice of me but needs must. After he'd left, I just up and told Tanya we needed to be together, but still she held out. To her, I could have anything and anyone I wanted, and she needed to know I wasn't just playing.

It was killing me. I'd been round for breakfast one day, but she'd quickly run off to get Kaley. I didn't know what to think.

So, it was time to find out. That night, I went around to see her again, and even though Joanne was there, I didn't care. I just blurted out, 'Do you see other boys?'

Who says that, really? 'Other boys'? What was I thinking? Tans should probably have made fun of me for pretending I was in some kind of terrible rom-com, but instead she simply said, 'No. I don't. I just want to be with you.'

Then there were three people in the room suddenly, and it was a bit awkward. But I didn't care.

'I want to be with you, too,' I said.

I was just glad Joanne didn't break out into applause or something.

Then, Tans said, 'I've got these butterflies inside me. It's making me behave strangely. I'm sorry.'

Tans didn't have to be sorry. Not at all.

From that day on I just wanted to spend every minute of god's waking day with her. Training was just getting in the way. But there was still one big hurdle: Mr Lou Lamont, Tanya's dad.

Lou is the epitome of an old-school guy – straighter than any arrow. At the time of Tans' and my marathon talking session, Lou had been away in Bournemouth, golfing, so he hadn't heard about what had happened. But it didn't take long for Tans and me to start spending more time together – in fact, the three women next door and the three of us lads at 5 Hunter's Oak spent all summer hanging out.

Later that summer, a friend of mine was throwing a wedding for his daughter and I'd been invited. This seemed like a great opportunity to take Tans on a real date. I asked her, but before she could commit to it, she told me she had to talk to her father. He was very much the head of the family: he organized everything, ran everything and everything went through him. He wasn't strict, per se, just straight – a stickler. There were the right ways to do things and the wrong ways. And, let's be honest, the right kind of people and the wrong. Tans was obviously worried that I'd be in the latter category.

But Tans was single-minded and when she wanted something, she wanted something – don't forget this is the girl who rode her horse down Gaddesden Crescent whenever she felt like it. So, she went to see her dad to fill him in on what was going on.

Tans started out carefully, telling Lou that she was going on a date. It was the first date she'd been on since splitting up with Steve, so it was a big deal. Naturally enough, Lou was interested in who it might be.

There was a long pause.

'Vincent Jones,' Tanya said – she always called me Vincent. But it didn't matter – Lou was able to work out who it was. At the time, my reputation was a national one, and let's just say it wasn't the best. There had been a few red cards and a few tackles that were notorious, shall we say.

Lou blew a gasket and went through the roof at the same time. 'Vinnie Jones? He's a nutter!' Lou shouted. 'You're not going out on a date with Vinnie Jones.'

But something about how Tanya looked, and what she said next, worked to bring him around.

'I've known him a long time,' Tanya said. 'He's the only man who's ever held a car door open for me. He's a perfect gentleman.' Tans was adamant.

Eventually Lou came around and okayed the date. He and I would become close (and remain so to this day); he comes over to the States a lot, and we play golf together, and I see him a lot back in the UK, now we're both without her. It's the one thing I wish we didn't share.

8

JOHNNY WATTS' DAUGHTER GETS MARRIED

But I'm rushing ahead again. First, I have to tell you what happened on our first date and let me just say up front that it involves a helicopter and a man singing 'War, what is it good for?'

At the time I still owned a house on St Agnells Lane in Hemel Hempstead, just around the corner from Hunter's Oak. There were a few bungalows further down on St Agnells, and one of them was owned by a guy called Johnny Watts. If he sounds like a character from a Paul Weller song or a Blur album then that's appropriate – he was larger than life was Johnny, a right old character, a gambler and a good-time Charley. All the lads used to go around to the bungalow and give Johnny the bets to go and put on at the bookies. We also used to see him in the pub and we loved him because he was just old school.

One day he grabbed me by the lapels at the bar.

'Vinnie my boy, my boy Vinnie,' Johnny said. 'My daughter is getting married and I'd like you to attend.' Then he said, 'We got everything. We've even got a helicopter . . .'

Nothing was beyond Johnny Watts; he didn't give a shit what anyone thought, and that was another reason why we loved him.

But St Agnells was a normal fucking street, so none of us had any idea how a helicopter would play into the plans. We couldn't wait to find out.

It was too good an opportunity to miss. I went around to see Tans and told her all about Johnny Watts and the coming nuptials.

'It's this bloke, Johnny Watts. Well, he's older than me . . .' I said, nervously. 'I mean, I've never met his daughter or anything,' I added, not making all that much sense. I don't know why I was so nervous. 'They're getting married,' I said, as though Johnny was marrying his daughter – did I mention I was nervous? 'He wants all the boys from the pub to go.'

Vinnie, just come out with it for Christ's sake.

'Would you come?' I finally said. 'Would you come with me? It'd be our first date.'

I was amazed Tans agreed (pending her chat with Lou, of course), given that it had taken me the best part of ten minutes to ask her. But for me, the pressure was off a bit – even though this was our first date on our own, I knew that all the lads from the pub and their wives and girlfriends would be going, so I'd be set if it didn't go too well.

The day of the wedding came, and honestly, I still can't believe what I saw.

Johnny had transformed his little bungalow on St Agnells

Lane into . . . well, into something, let me tell you. He'd put in artificial ponds all around the garden, and you had to walk over a bridge to get to the other side. It was bizarre. He'd also put a massive marquee up at the back which he'd managed to attach to the back of his house; there were drapes everywhere, too, and chandeliers hanging from the top. And we also noticed he'd taken his back fence down, so that you could now walk straight out of the marquee, over the bridge and the ponds, trailing your hand along the satin drapes if you so wished, and out onto the football pitch that adjoined his property to the rear.

As one sage put it as we arrived, 'What the fuck?'

The party was in full swing, and we were all sitting round at a table. I was proudly introducing Tans as my date and everyone was amazed. 'Fucking hell, Jonesy, are you sure?' They knew I was punching way over my class.

'Yeah, fucking yeah,' I said, 'don't worry about it, lads.' Everyone knew I'd sworn off marriage, or even a serious relationship, so this was news: Vinnie Jones had a girlfriend.

But we were having a great night. People were coming by to say hello – I was the Babycham guy, that night.

They were amazed I was with a date, finally. Up till then, I'd been very happy to just rock and roll with the boys. I loved men's company; I had to be in the pub after training, had to have the lads live at my house. Most days we had the crash on . . . so for me to have brought a date? This was news.

'Oh, you must be special because he doesn't usually have

one on his arm,' one of my mates told Tans. 'He's never brought anyone to one of the dos.'

One of the wives agreed. 'He's never brought one out,' she said, as though she'd seen a UFO.

I looked at Tans and said, 'This is my family, Tans, you know?'

And she knew; she always knew. She was having a great time, too; the craic was mighty that night. And Tans looked so beautiful – she was wearing a little white, cotton, lacy dress, just above the knee. Awesome.

After a few hours, I believed I'd nailed it with her. We were about to leave – I didn't want to stay for the sloppy punch-up and all the rest of it. It had been too great. But as we were preparing our goodbyes, all of a sudden Johnny Watts came over.

'Vinnie my boy!' he shouted. He loved the celebrity stuff and I was playing for Chelsea at the time, so I was a favourite of his.

'We're about to do the laser thing, Vin,' Watts said. 'You just watch this.'

All the lads were laughing. 'This is all to impress you, Vinnie,' someone said.

Just then, the laser show began. The music started and we heard 'Eye to eye contact' and it's the actual, real-to-goodness, Edwin fucking Starr. In a marquee, on St Agnells Lane, Hemel Hempstead, singing:

If she raised her head her eyes caught mine
And that was all that I needed

In her eyes I saw the need for love
The warm, soft feeling
'Cause we made, eye to eye contact

Tans said, 'Edwin Starr?'

I said, 'Just a regular Saturday night, love.'

It doesn't get any better than that. Until it does. Never had the words of that song sounded so exciting and electric.

Once Starr had finished his set, Johnny took the microphone and made a grand announcement.

'Everybody outside, the bride and groom are leaving!' he intoned. We all trooped out, and there, out on the public football pitch beyond his house, we all watched, gobsmacked, as a helicopter appeared out of the dark night. And it was then we realized that it was preparing to land.

Only Johnny Watts could do this. People up and down St Agnells Street were freaking out but Johnny didn't care – things were a bit different then. He'd never asked anyone; he'd just taken the fence down and brought in a helicopter because this was his daughter's big day and she deserved the best. The bride and groom walked out of the marquee, across the bridges over the ponds and, ducking, headed into the helicopter, whose blades continued to whirl in the Hemel Hempstead night.

The entire party had moved out to the football pitch to watch the scene. I pulled Tans into me, standing behind her with my arms around her shoulders. She leaned into me and we settled there, perfectly content, perfectly fitting into each other, at ease, as though we'd known each other forever – which in a way I suppose we had. We were surrounded by everyone from the wedding, but we were alone together. It was the most perfect moment you can imagine.

The blades whirred harder, the grass shook, dust flew around and the helicopter started to wobble just above the ground, then steadily climb. Everyone around us cheered and waved. I pulled Tans even closer to me and we watched this great whirlybird rise up into the dark night, its lights getting dimmer and the sound of the engines fading until it was just a faint shudder in the sky. And then it was gone; the bride and groom in their helicopter were gone and we don't know how long we've been standing there, watching this hilarious and ridiculous and touching thing, this magical moment at the start of two people's lives together . . .

When we finally came back to earth, when we finally woke from that dream into which we'd fallen, we looked around and realized we were alone. Everyone else had gone back into the marquee to dance to whatever people dance to at weddings. We had been so wrapped up in each other that we hadn't noticed, not at all, that we were the only ones left. The helicopter had flown and we had stood together, perfectly still in the new knowledge of each other; we had gelled instantly, welded together like two people who'd finally found home.

Tans said, 'Oh, that was so lovely.'

I said, 'That's going to be us one day.' And it was.

*

About a year after that amazing night, I remember Tans asking me, 'What do you want from me? What can I give you?'

And I just said to her, 'I just want to be loved, because I've been in turmoil.'

My old man has often said, 'You had a great childhood – look at the life I gave you.' But honestly, my childhood was fucked. From 15 years old I was living on people's couches – Tanya knew the story because I'd told her that first long night at Hunter's Oak. Although we didn't know it then, we were falling in love with each other that very first night – in retrospect it felt like we had been taking our vows. When I had told her about my childhood, Tans had burst into tears: 'How could this happen to you?' she said.

And finally, when Tans said, 'What do you want?' I found myself saying, 'I just need to be loved unconditionally.' She was the only person on the planet who could do that for me. She understood it; she understood what I needed. And it never wavered. Much, much later, whatever Tanya was doing, wherever she was – if she was out somewhere in England, or having fun around L.A – even if she was having a whale of a time, she'd tell everyone, 'We've got to get back. Vin doesn't like coming home to an empty house.' Tans knew what I'd been through, the fights and the couch-es and the emptiness and the loneliness and not knowing where my next 'home' was going to be. And she was never going to have me come home to an empty house. That was the promise she made.

Today, six months after she's gone, I came home to an empty house. I sat in the living room, on my expensive couch in my lovely L.A. house, and even though I could feel her all around me, and even though I had one of my little chats with her, I knew deep down that I would always come home to an empty house. I felt a chill then, even though it was 24 degrees out; a deep, bone-deep chill, as though I was sick.

But I wasn't sick. I was just alone again.

The hardest part of it now is that I've gone full circle; an empty house is all I'll ever come home to. Kaley has been amazing – she's really stepped up to keep the family together and to look after me – but she won't live with me forever . . .

But something interesting has happened too: for the first time in my life, I am genuinely OK with being alone. I think that's because I've got Tans with me, everywhere I go. In the old days, everyone would say, 'Oh, Vin always has to have a gang with him.' But not anymore.

I'm just back from a short promotional tour. I did four nights – Watford to Leeds, Leeds to Sheffield – 700 miles in four days. Before I lost Tans, I would have had a driver for a trip like that and a couple of mates with me, too, probably. But this time I did all the driving on my own; I think it's because that was my time with Tans. I feel she's with me. I have my little thought chats with her, and the time passes, and before I know it, I'm bounding out on stage singing a Madness song.

The thought chats make all the difference. She's everywhere with me. Not like an angel, or a spirit, but a real presence, in the air, in the sounds the air makes, in the way the light falls across a couch or the floor, that floor right there. See?

Tanya and Shane —
sister and brother, and
best friends all her life.

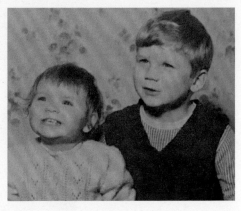

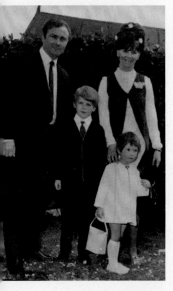

Tanya and Shane with their parents,
Lou and Maureen Lamont. Tans was
already a fashion maven, even by the
age of three.

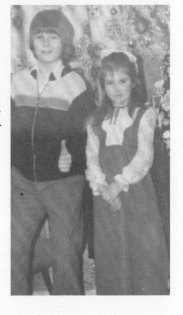

Shane pretending to run for prime
minister? Tanya would have voted for
him — she was his biggest fan.

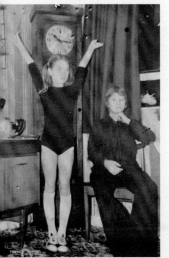

Tanya and Shane at Ganders Ash, in front
of a clock that's still there. Tanya wore
that leotard at all times so she could do her
gymnastics at a moment's notice.

Tans was beautiful inside and out. I was so punching above my weight — and that's a feeling I had until the day she died.

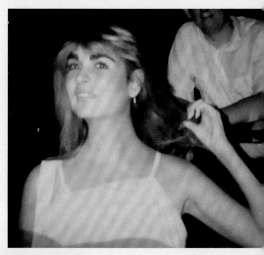

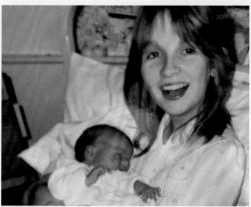

In Watford General, right after having Kaley, and right before her heart stopped working.

Tans couldn't have known that in a few weeks she'd receive a heart transplant that would save her life.

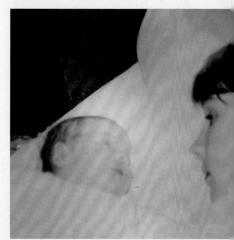

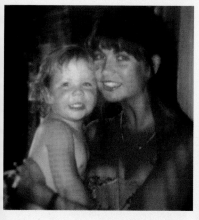

Summers at Hunter's Oak with Kaley.
I moved in next door by chance,
and the rest is history.

Tans loved being a mother;
she and Kaley shared an
otherworldly bond.

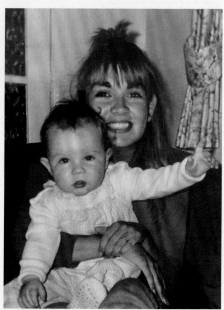

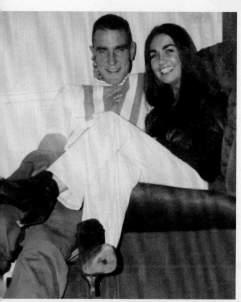

My first Christmas as a
guest of Lou and Maureen
at Gaddesden Crescent.

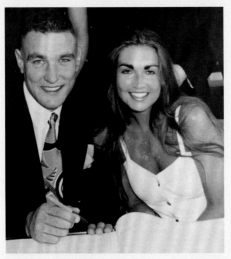

We loved each other so much we got married twice; once in a registry office on Friday, 24 June 1994, and again on Saturday, 25 June 1994 at our house at Redbourn.

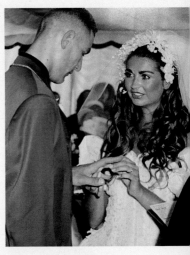

For our Saturday wedding 200 people attended the ceremony, and 400 came to the party in the evening.

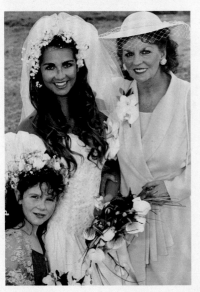

With her mum, Maureen, and Kaley.

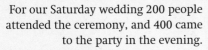

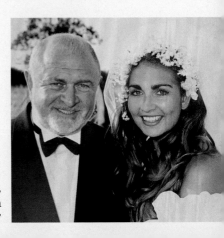

In Lou's father-of-the-bride speech, he said, 'Vinnie has a heart problem too — it's too big for his body.'

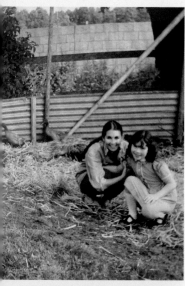

At Redbourn we had eight chickens and two cockerels, a pair of ducks, a couple of ferrets, a rabbit, two Vietnamese pot-bellied pigs, two peacocks and a ton of dogs. It was heaven.

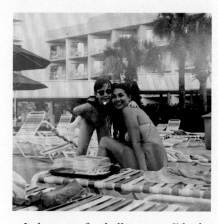

In between football seasons, I'd take Kaley and Tans on holiday — here we are in Florida, with chicken strips and chips for lunch.

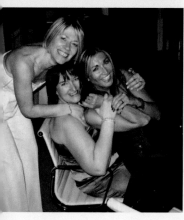

With two of her dearest friends, Jo Southern (standing) and Julie McGregor, on Tans' fortieth birthday at The Grove in Watford.

Tans always loved to ride. Her dad, Lou, had gotten her a horse (Persephone) when she was young — here they are riding together years later in Griffith Park in Los Angeles.

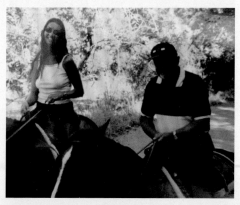

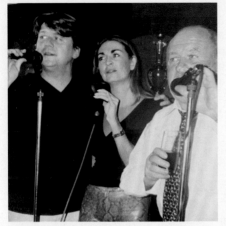

Music was a big part of our lives together — Shane never played his guitar in pubs and restaurants or at parties without seeing his sister singing along to every word. Here they are with their dad on a karaoke night.

My beautiful, sweet, funny, kind, tough, modest, loving Tanya.

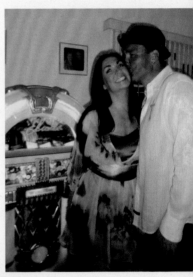

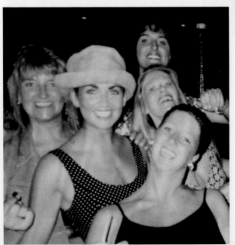

Tans was the centre of everything for so many people.

We cleaned up OK — with Maureen, Tans' mum.

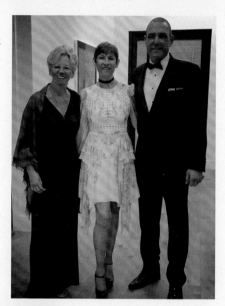

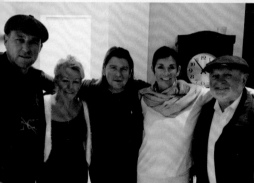

Me, Maureen, Shane, Tans and Lou — on Tans' last-ever visit to the UK. (That's the same clock from the leotard photo.)

Just a few months before she died, Tans wanted to go to Venice Beach in Los Angeles, where she'd always get a henna tattoo that said, 'I love Vin'. Here she is linking arms with Kaley, determined to have a special day out with her daughter.

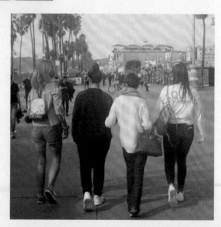

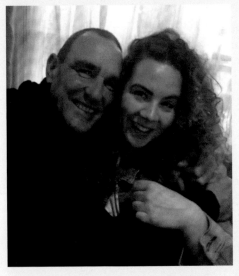

Tans took this picture of me and Kaley. Our job now is to look after each other as best we can. That was Tans' wish.

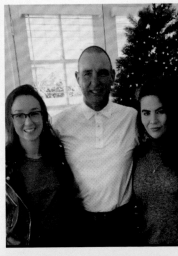

With Kaley and Lauren, at our last Christmas with Tans.

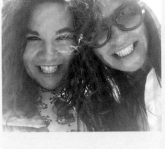

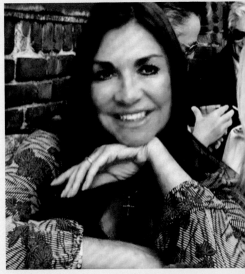

Tanya and Kaley were inseparable. Tanya always told Kaley she was her 'life's most precious gift'. Kaley now says the same about Tanya.

9

WHAT HAPPENED IN NUNEATON

At 3 Hunter's Oak, Tanya worked on getting back to full health. After she and Steve had split, Tans had decided to create a lovely home filled with a whole bunch of mums to her Kaley. There was Jo, Julie, Jane, and Mandy – Kaley loved Jane the most back then, because when she was a kid she thought Jane was the coolest. Julie was the sensible one – she would sometimes go around and try and help Tans learn how to grocery shop on a budget, all that. Remember, Tans was a baby, and was in charge of a little nipper who asked for stuff. Kaley vividly remembers desperately wanting some Matey's Bubble Bath – the one with the sailor's hat for a top – but Julie said it was too expensive and mum needed to be firm with her. (Tans got it for her anyway.)

The gang would order an Indian or Chinese and sit around the table putting the world to rights over a glass of wine. There were endless games of Frustration, and so much laughter.

That was why when I arrived at the door late that fateful night, Kaley called out for her mum – Kaley hated being left out if there was fun to be had downstairs. Usually, the girls would take it in turns to go up and check on Kaley – sometimes Kaley would lock Jane in the cupboard because she didn't want her to go back downstairs.

Tans was the only one of the gang who had a child. The rest were all single or starting to date – usually one of my mates, actually. The two houses side-by-side on Hunter's Oak must have looked from the outside like a cliched version of those TV shows of the nineties, the ones where in the summer the boys are doing the gardening with their tops off and rocking the washed-out jeans, then the camera pans to find all the girls passing by on roller skates.

Tans was just a few years past her transplant, but nothing stopped her living a normal life. It was clear she'd decided to just get on with it. She would take Kaley to the amusement park at Chessington or Alton Towers and, once, to Disneyland. Everywhere they walked in those places there were big signs saying:

PERSONS WITH THE FOLLOWING CONDITIONS SHOULD NOT RIDE:
Heart Conditions or Abnormal Blood Pressure

According to Kaley, though, Tans just ignored the warnings and rode everything she could – she'd be hysterically laughing the whole time and Kaley would just stare at her like she'd lost her mind.

Sometimes, too, all the girls would go and watch Shane play music. He'd moved to the States for a while in his twenties and when he came back he would play all those Laurel Canyon songs – the Jackson Browne stuff, the Graham Nash stuff – in pubs and restaurants and clubs around Watford. But Shane never sang a note without his adoring sister in the front row, singing along to every single word. Tans was his biggest fan, she was so proud of him up there doing his thing. It was like she was born with an overflow of love, too much for one person.

Because Kaley knew all about the transplant, she would accompany Tans to every appointment, at least early on. Whenever Kaley was at Harefield, she got some sad comfort from the fact that she'd see people there who looked a lot sicker than her mum did. They even had a club for the transplant patients called 'The Hamster Club', because you puff out after you have a transplant – though Tans hated it and never wanted to be part of it. She didn't look like a transplant recipient; she looked healthy and strong (though her skin darkened after the surgery – no one ever knew why).

These would be long days for the two of them. Tans called it 'clinic', as in, 'we have clinic today', and she and Kaley would go through all the tests together. These involved Tans having her bloods drawn and getting weighed and doing stress tests. Kaley remembers her mum laughing and being happy and cuddly, always making sure that her daughter felt safe and not scared. And then there was the long wait for the results, until she'd finally get to see Dr Mitchell and he'd give her the good news.

But on a day-to-day basis, Tans was just living a normal

life – and then some. Tans would go into the garden with Kaley and I'd watch her show her all the gymnastics moves she knew, right there on the summer lawn, her second heart working just fine, her limbs all lithe and strong – a brilliant athlete, she was. She was basically a fit young woman . . . until she wasn't. There was one birthday in particular when Kaley had wanted to go to a Spice Girls concert, but her mum hadn't been feeling too great, so Julie and Mandy took her (though part of me wonders if Tans felt fine and just didn't fancy the Spice Girls).

There were other times when Tans' health affected their lives. She had to be very careful about which pets were allowed in the house. George the rabbit had been banished to the shed because he was a danger to Tans' health; puppies were OK, but birds were not because of the diseases they can carry, so it was no parrots. Kaley desperately wanted a monkey – a monkey in Hemel Hempstead would have been brilliant, of course – but Tans had to say no.

As for me and Tanya, well, things were going great. We were in love but we were still finding our way through the relationship . . . that is, until Tans had to go up to Nuneaton for a minor operation.

The heavy drugs Tans had to take took their toll and led to her needing a partial hysterectomy. I didn't pry into what exactly was going on but I knew it was serious and it scared her; she'd already been through so much, this felt unfair, somehow.

Tans headed the 80 miles up the M1 to have her operation

and I missed her every second. I hated not being with her (that wouldn't change in 27 years). Her friends Mandy and Jo had gone with her, so she was set for support and visitors, but it didn't feel right. Already, I think, I looked at Tans as a member of my family. You know that feeling when you meet someone and instantly their needs are your needs? Or you feel so in tune with them that you don't settle until they're OK? Well, that was me and Tans, very soon after we'd reconnected.

One day I'd been training at Chelsea when I got a call from Mandy. She told me that the doctors wanted to keep Tans in after her operation for a few days so they could monitor her; I think whenever any doctor heard about the transplant, they were extra careful.

Then Mandy put Tans on the phone. Her voice was tiny, far away, scared: 'Vincent,' she said, 'will you come and get me?'

My heart sank and filled at the same time. I felt so sorry for how sad and scared Tans sounded and I wanted to fix it, right there and then. Nearly 20 years later I'd tell Angela Levin of the *Daily Mail*:

> I take my strength from Tanya. She believes her life was saved to save me, and in return I feel it is my role to look after her and give her the best life I can.
>
> She has given me stability and it is my responsibility to be there for her. When we are apart, I make sure she is never on her own.
>
> Goodness knows where I would be without her.

But those words were true in 1992 when she called me from her hospital bed in Nuneaton.

I'm surprised I wasn't nicked on the M1 to be honest. Let's just say that if you were driving north sometime in 1992 and a Range Rover passed you doing at least a ton, I'm sorry.

Unbeknownst to me, Tanya was preparing for my arrival. She had borrowed some makeup from the nurses and had dolled herself up for me. She really was an amazing person. (Kaley always says to me, 'Mum was this really positive, loving, happy person who didn't seem any different to anyone else.') So there she was, lying in her hospital bed, her lippy shining, her hair all done up; she looked so beautiful. The second I saw her I was determined to get her out of there, immediately – well, she'd asked, for a start!

The doctors, though, weren't having it. After a whole bunch of back and forth, they weren't budging; Tans had to stay a few more days until they were sure everything was OK.

Sorry, lads, but no. I was not leaving without her – not in a million years, not if you paid me a million quid. There was only one thing for it. I gave her the eye and she beamed back at me. Then I pulled back the covers, wrapped her in one of the hospital blankets and did the full *An Officer and a Gentlemen* thing – I picked her up and, with the doctors complaining and the nurses quietly cheering, I carried her out of the hospital in my arms and laid her on the rear seat of my car.

Jo and Mandy couldn't believe it, but I didn't care; she was coming home with me.

And yes, I'd thought ahead: there were pillows and a duvet back there, so she'd be comfortable. Jo and Mandy brought all the flowers she'd been sent, and we put them all around the car. Then very gingerly I drove south, hardly breaking 40mph this time, all the while telling her she was going to be fine.

Later, when her dad heard the story, I think he realized I was in it for the long haul, which was a good thing. Remember, nationally I had a bit of a reputation by 1992. In 1987, I'd grabbed Gazza by his meat and two veg; there had been a few red cards since then, shall we say, and perhaps some tackles that might have warranted more than a yellow or a talking to (here's looking at you, McMahon). The *Soccer's Hard Men* video came out in 1992 – the one in which I extolled the virtues of football thuggery, and for which my old mate Sam Hammam had amusingly called me 'a mosquito brain'. I'd been fined twenty grand and banned for six months by the F.A. for it (though the ban had been a suspended one, and I played on).

But when Lou heard I'd sprung Tans from hospital, driven her home, and then looked after her for the next few days, I think he thought, *hold on a minute* . . .

I didn't do it for effect, though. I did it because finally I was able to fully love someone and show them that love in a real and concrete way. It felt natural, and right. That was us, right there – sorted. We honestly never looked back. It felt like *Gulliver's Travels* – two big giants had been put on the planet and been told, 'go find each other'.

And we did, right there on the M1, 40 m.p.h. on the inside lane, driving south from beautiful Nuneaton in a car filled with flowers.

One day, Tans was out picking up Kaley from school and I decided to make a shepherd's pie for when they got back. I remember needing a spatula to spread out the mashed potato on top and I couldn't find one. There was one drawer I hadn't looked in, but it wouldn't open – it was jammed with something. I tugged and tugged and managed to pry it free, only to see that it was filled with red letters from the electric, the gas, the TV, everyone. I knew she was a bit short of cash, but this was something else. I knew what I had to do – I ran around to my house next door, got my chequebook and I just wrote a whole load of cheques.

When Tans got back, I told her what I'd done, and I said, 'I'm taking care of all this now; I'm moving in.' Tans tried to make a joke of it – 'Well, they just kept sending these red letters – were they just trying to scare me?' But we knew this was a watershed moment for our relationship.

I didn't make a fuss of it. Instead, I got the shepherd's pie out of the oven, dished it up and the three of us – Tanya, Kaley and Vin, a new family – sat there eating it and grinning from ear to ear.

10

DING DONG THE BELLS ARE GONNA CHIME

I didn't have a moment to waste: I had to marry Tanya.

I felt a love that I hadn't felt for a long, long time. I hadn't seen much of my mum; she had moved to live in a bedsit in a nursing home, and it was hard to see her for a while – it just didn't feel natural. I'd fallen out with the old man, too; I didn't have much to do with him after he punched me through a window. I just think I hadn't had a lot of love. I had moved in with a big local family, John and Wendy Moore and their four kids, when I was 18, and I mostly stayed with them for the next five years.

By the time I moved to play for Leeds the old man came back on the scene and he came to all the games, but when I went to Sheffield United, he didn't come as much because we were losing – 'I don't want to watch that shit,' he'd say.

Tans knew all this. She said to me, 'What's missing? What?' She's the only person ever to ask me that. 'What's missing? What can I do? What do you want from me?' It was probably one of the first times I'd been honest with anybody for a long, long time, and I just said, 'I want you to unconditionally love me.' Just like in the movies.

And Tanya just threw her arms around me and said, 'Forever and ever and ever.'

One day, Tans and me were stood looking over the garden to see Kaley in a toy electric Jeep we'd bought her, driving around with Aaron, who was about one or two, in the passenger seat.

I never ever thought I'd get married – I was going to be single for the rest of my life. But out there in the garden those two little dots were bonding in a toy car, and in the house, Tans and I stood watching, filled with love for them and for each other. See why I didn't have a minute to waste?

So now marriage was all I wanted, and I really needed to tell someone. The next day I was in my full-size car, and I called my father.

He picked up and said, 'How you doing, son?'

I said, 'I'm going to ask Tanya to marry me.'

He said, 'Oh, wow. Yeah, OK. Anyway, I've been up to the house and fed the pheasants . . .' And that was that. All I could do was drive around, on my own as ever.

I decided to drive to see Lou. By then, he and I had started to play golf a bit and become closer. On the way to Lou's, I called another friend of mine to tell him what I was planning, but his reaction was even worse than my dad's – he said, 'It won't last six months.' I was very hurt and made sure he wasn't invited to the wedding. (I've seen the guy since, actually, a few years ago, and he apologized. I said, 'Why would you say something like that?' and he just said, 'I didn't think she'd put up with you!')

When I arrived at Lou's, I got straight to the point. 'I want to ask Tans if I can marry her,' I said.

Lou was concerned about his daughter's health issues. He said, 'Listen son, you know she's not an ordinary girl? It's going to be a tough road.'

I said, 'I think that's what I'm here for. I think that's my duty. I think that's what it's all about. I will look after her.'

And Lou believed me. And I looked after her, as I'd promised, for the rest of her life.

Meanwhile, Tans was waiting at home for me to be done with asking everyone's permission except hers. She knew it was coming.

When I got home, I carried her upstairs and put her on the bed. I even remembered to take her shoes off . . . and then I'd knelt down by the bed and asked her.

Tans burst into tears; this was not a good sign.

'What are you crying for?' I said, worried half to death.

'What took you so long?' Tans said.

We were married on Friday 24 June 1994, and again on Saturday 25 June 1994. That can happen when you're trying to avoid the press. First, you head to the registry office on Clarendon Road in Watford to do the paperwork and then the next day you have a massive blow-out affair and take your vows in your new house.

Right before we got married, I'd bought us an old farmstead in Redbourn, ten minutes up the road from Hunters Oak. I wanted a place that was ours and ours alone; a place where Kaley could run around free and where Aaron could visit whenever he wanted. And I wanted somewhere where

Tans could watch the spring and summer arrive in the skies and in the fields. She loved the sun so much and she'd overcome so much . . . I wanted the best for her and the farm at Redbourn was a first step.

When we bought it, the place was a falling-down two-bedroom bungalow lived in by some travellers. Me and my old man took a year to rebuild it and we finished it the day before the wedding. It was perfect. The landscaping, the fixtures, the gardens – all finished just in time for hundreds of people to descend on it and celebrate with us as Mr White, the local vicar, blessed the union.

We were also blessed by the tabloids. We sold the Saturday wedding to the *News of the World* – they paid £100,000, which was a lot of dough in 1994. I didn't care that it was all 'Beauty and the Beast' stuff; I knew where our hearts were. What the *News of the World* cared about was their investment, though, so they brought cardboard boxes to shield the whole thing from other paparazzi and even from helicopters that were circling, trying to get pictures. There was one road in and out of Redbourn and the *News of the World* blocked it off, making it hard for all the guests to get through. At one point, I had to jump a wall to avoid the paps after the registry office ceremony. Tans was surrounded by all her friends to keep her secret, too.

The night before, I had my stag do at the Aubrey Park Hotel while Tans and her girls were back at the house. The morning of the wedding, Tans went to a local café with all her mates, her rollers still in, to have breakfast – that's how down to earth she was. There were 200 people present for the Saturday ceremony and 400 in the evening.

It was hot as hell that day. What I didn't know was that Tans could barely walk; the medication she was on for her heart had the terrible side effect of giving her gout. She was in agony; her mum even called Dr Mitchell at Harefield and he called in a prescription to the chemist on Garston Parade (she would get her drugs there throughout her life).

In his speech, Lou said something special: 'Vinnie has a heart problem too – it's too big for his body.'

(Later, Tans would tell *OK!* magazine, 'He's the most emotional man I've ever met. He sometimes wakes me up in the middle of the night just to tell me he loves me. He worries about me a lot and he is great in a crisis. He holds me so tight he almost crushes me.')

It was a great wedding, even though Tans was in so much pain that she had to go and buy bigger shoes that very morning just so she could walk. We made everyone give a donation to Harefield instead of presents.

At the end of the night we left in a helicopter, as promised, and went to Juan-les-Pins, half-way between Cannes and Nice, because Peter Sarstedt's 'Where Do You Go To My Lovely?' was our favourite tune and that's one of the places the character goes in the song.

But it wasn't to be the last time that a helicopter would come to Redbourn, and next time it wasn't anywhere near as romantic.

11

HE TOOK ONE THROUGH
THE WINDOW

On the field, I'd left Chelsea and returned to Wimbledon; I would play another six years there.

My day off from Wimbledon was Tuesday, and I'd fill each of them with hunting, fishing and, I'm sorry to say, drinking. One Tuesday in November 1997, three years after we'd got married, I awoke to a late autumn day that would turn into a beauty: sunny and 11 degrees. I'd rushed out to do what I loved the most – tracking pheasants across the fields.

Buying the farm and doing it up had been a dream come true. This was a farm that had been there since the end of the thirteenth century and was famous in the county. We, on the other hand, were just two kids from solidly working-class backgrounds: Tans grew up on a Gaddesden estate, and my house was adjacent to a council estate, Bedmond, and that's where all my friends lived and where I hung out. We never dreamed, either of us, that we'd one day own a three-acre plot at the end of a dirt track.

I was determined to make it magical, especially for the kids, so I bought every kind of animal. But, to be honest, it spiralled out of control a bit. For a start, we had eight chickens and two cockerels, a pair of ducks and a couple of ferrets and a rabbit, of course. Then there were the two Vietnamese pot-bellied pigs – Kaley named them Pete and Dud. Only problem was, at the time I wasn't an expert pig sexer (I'm still not), so I missed the fact that they were gilts – females. Which would have been fine, except I also thought it would be fun to have a boar – him I called Horace. Well, as the world turns, so the thoughts of pigs will turn to love, and soon I had piglets coming out of my ears.

It felt like we had magic dust sprinkled on us every day.

Then there were the peacocks. What's a country farm without a pair of peacocks? There was a pet store a couple of miles from the farm and one day they had two peacocks for sale. Done, bosh. Now we were the proud owners of two beautiful birds, which we named Elvis and Priscilla. One day soon after, Kaley came running into the kitchen heartbroken: there was no sign of Elvis and Priscilla. I honestly never thought they'd fly away; we fed them berries and grain and the odd insect – we even gave them livestock feed, which is like the best French food for a peacock. Why would they fly away when they were being treated to five-course cuisine at Chez Jones?

But I wasn't having Kaley be so upset; we were a little family now and she already meant the world to me. So I jumped in the car and went back to the pet store; luckily, they had two other peacocks, so I bought them, hoping it would make up for the loss of Elvis and Priscilla.

And, just like the first two, these peacocks got the best of everything: I even gave them a bit more livestock feed so they wouldn't be tempted to fly off. Well bugger me if a couple of weeks later there was no sign of them! What was I doing wrong? They were living like prince and princesses ... Back to the store, two more peacocks, livestock feed, Kaley happy, bosh.

Two more weeks, no peacocks. By now I was pretty much done with this malarkey, but Kaley and Tans loved those birds, and I have to say when they displayed their feathers it was a sight to see. But I told Kaley this was the last time I was replacing them. Peacocks aren't cheap – it was costing me around two hundred quid every time. The owner of the store, of course, was very happy to see me, though he must have thought I had a weird peafowl fetish or something.

Driving home, I had a nagging feeling in my brain, with the peacocks in the back staring at me as I drove. They seemed a bit smug to be honest ... not to mention *familiar*. And then it struck me: these fuckers were Elvis and Priscilla and had been all along. They were just flying back to the store and I'd go and drop another two hundred quid to repatriate them.

Clever sods, peacocks (and pet store owners).

But I didn't really mind because it was a little bit of heaven for all of us, but especially for Kaley and Aaron – we'd send her out to get the eggs every day, and they had motorbikes and quad bikes and a swimming pool and all the animals. When I was there, Kaley always called me Vin, but when I wasn't around – off at training or a game or some-where – Tans told me she referred to me as 'Dad'. She'd say to Tans, 'Where's Dad tonight?' or, 'Is Dad playing this weekend?' I can't tell you how much that meant to me, and still does.

Kaley quickly became as protective of me as her mum was. And I like to think that I was her safety net too, like I was for Tans. That's not going to change, not for a second. That's part of me honouring her mother's life. Kaley was everything to Tans.

Kaley loved Redbourn; we all did. At night, once she was asleep, Tans and I would lie in bed watching TV and having a cuddle, listening to the barn owl screeching in the woods. Each time I left the house to go somewhere, Tans would say, 'Where's my kiss?' and I'd throw her one – I'd literally throw her a kiss and she'd catch it.

But even our love couldn't save me that night, as the helicopters circled.

We were one of three properties on the acreage. There was our farmhouse, then another farmhouse at the bottom of the hill and a mobile home between the two.

Back then, I'd tried to help out an old homeless fella called Bill. He was 67, toothless and a drinker, and he used to hang around outside the Bell and Shears pub on the main drag in Redbourn. He wasn't in great shape, so one evening I offered to let him live in his tent in our field – in return, his job was to walk the dogs and do other stuff around the farm.

I was a bit of a sucker for dogs (still am). I think people knew that, so quite often on Sundays, people would come by not-so-randomly to the Bell and Shears and tell me a long sob story about this dog or that dog – they were usually working animals like shepherds and spaniels and Labradors – and how they needed a home. Those big eyes (of the dogs, not the owners) would gaze up at me and bosh, I'd head home with yet another animal. Quite a few nights I'd run upstairs to where Kaley was in bed and deposit a new dog on her duvet.

'Here's Sally!' I'd say one week, then the next week, 'Here's Taffy!' There was Ben the Alsatian – he got nicked – and Billy, the mutt. Most of these dogs we kept outside in the kennels and Bill would feed them and look after them. Two Jack Russells lived in the house, though – a mother and son team called Tessie and Lucky.

This acquisition of animals went on until I upped my game and brought home a human, Bill. We quickly converted a normal garden shed for him so that he'd have heating and electricity – not to mention Sky TV. Then, after the shed, I bought him a beautiful, all-singing, all-dancing caravan. We put it in the pig field and Tans used to do his dinner every night. Every single night. She was up for everything, our Tans; the kindest soul you can imagine.

I was forever bringing something home to Redbourn. One Bonfire Night I brought back an entire set of fairground rides that I'd borrowed from some Travellers, complete with carousels and hot dog stands, the lot. Bouncy castles became a regular thing too, so that all the neighbourhood kids could have fun with Kaley and Aaron.

Then there were the little business schemes I ran. I was on good money from the football, but I still liked to dabble.

The first thing I got into was TVs. I bought 150 of them at £125 a pop and then I'd sell them for two hundred. I think they were Russian rejects, Bekos, from Argos, and I kept them in the garage. You couldn't get a mouse in there, there were so many TVs in boxes. Sadly, we found out after I sold them that none of them worked. People would bring them back and I'd replace them with a different Beko, which was also no good. I tried to take the whole lot back to the guy I'd gotten them from, but he said, 'The rules are: bought as seen.' I didn't like to point out that technically that was just *one* rule, and honestly, he wasn't the kind of person to argue with, so I didn't press the point.

From broken TVs I graduated to nesting tables; I thought they'd be a lovely Christmas gift for wives and mothers and girlfriends. Who doesn't love a set of mahogany nesting tables? On Christmas Day, however, my phone lit up like a Christmas tree, because when the lads all proudly presented their lady folk with the nesting tables, each and every one had a leg missing (the tables, not the ladies). I had some tables left over so I could at least get a few spare legs from the unused boxes, but it still wasn't a good look.

My last foray into merchandise was toasters. I bought a

job lot for six quid each, sold them for a tenner. I bought 200 of them; nothing could go wrong this time.

Well. My mate had just decorated his mum's kitchen all white, beautiful. To finish off the look, my mate had paid me a tenner for a toaster. One morning, his mum put the bread in and it was Bonfire Night all over again. Bang, wallop, the bread flew up in a spray of sparks all the way up to the new white ceiling. There were burn marks and black shit everywhere. It seems the toasters hadn't been wired correctly; I heard a few houses got fried, a few fuses blown here and there.

But Tans thought it was as hilarious as I did. She always stood by me, even when things went bang, or when TVs didn't work, or when furniture resembled the Leaning Nesting Tables of Pisa. She'd never say, when are you going to learn your lesson? She just knew I loved all that shit, the wheeling and dealing, the craic.

A year or two after we got married, I was driving back from training to Redbourn when I got a call from the Arsenal boys – Tony Adams, Ray Parlour, Paul Merson and John Hartson. They were at the Watersplash Hotel in London Colney, which they knew was just up the road from Redbourn, about 10 miles. And that's all it took. 'Alright, I'm on my way,' I said – M25, bosh, do me lovely. I arrived at about half past two in the afternoon ... and somehow didn't leave until eight o'clock the next morning. Card games had led to more card games had led to me calling up my mates and neighbours in Redbourn and in the end everyone turned up.

It wasn't as bad as the time I went to the races at Sandown one morning and woke up the next morning in fucking Dublin and had no idea how I got there. I remember looking at the phone in the hotel, seeing the Irish code on it and thinking, 'What the fuck?' But it wasn't good, all the same. When I drank, I drank, and there were too often consequences to pay. That was the problem with my drinking: I was a binge drinker and I just made terrible decisions.

One such bad decision was to take the Arsenal lads back with me to Redbourn in a black cab, figuring, unwisely, that there might be eggs and bacon in the offing. We all sort of bounced out of the cab and there was Tans, just taking Kaley to school. She took one look at me, slammed the car door and drove past us at high speed. We dived out of the way and Basil, my mate down the road, said, 'I'm off. I ain't going to be here when she gets home.'

When she got home, things were a bit ... frosty, shall we say, for a couple of days at least. But I didn't sleep on the couch – she would always wake me to go to bed with her, always, and that night was no exception, even though there had been no dinner. She knew I'd slept on couches as a kid and she hated sleeping alone too, so however mad she was – and with good reason – I never woke up on the couch in my own home. And I always knew when she was mad because her voice would get higher pitched. She may have thought herself a lovely farm girl from *Little House on the Prairie*, but cross her and the tough girl from Garston would show up.

After the Arsenal night, Kaley reckons I probably got

Tans a card. And even though there was no dinner the first night, the next night maybe I got a little bit of something, and eventually things settled out. It never took too long because we never believed we had too long. We knew deep down that life was going to be short for us, although you stick your head in the sand about it. But still, we sort of agreed that we didn't have time to not talk to each other for a week.

Tans would stick up for me in so many ways. Sometimes it was comical – even I couldn't stick up for myself for some of the things I did, but she'd be there, backing me up.

I was lucky enough to play nine times for Wales; the players even voted me captain, which probably pissed Bobby Gould off (he was the manager). Needless to say, even though I'd learned the Welsh national anthem from Gary Speed (god rest his soul) and put my heart into it, I still managed to screw up.

In June 1995, after about half an hour of a game against Georgia in the Euros qualifying rounds, I stamped on one of the Georgia players and was sent off. As soon as I stamped on the guy, I remember thinking, 'Why? What are you doing? No need for it, no need whatsoever.' Back at the hotel, Maureen, Lou and Tans and everyone were waiting for me, and Tans just said, 'Well, he shouldn't have been lying there, should he?'

Two years later, I tested her patience in a much more serious way at Redbourn.

*

141

We heard the helicopters before we saw them.

I was standing at the kitchen sink, running my bloodied knuckles under the tap. I'd really done it this time. Tans was looking at me with a mixture of fear and anger, but mostly I could tell she was starting to get really scared; in fact, she was hyperventilating.

This was the bit I always hated. I could handle myself; I'd had a hundred fights; I'd been arrested; I'd done some overnights in the custody of Her Majesty's; I knew how to deal with the Old Bill, all that. But Tans hated it. *Hated* it. It was the look on her face I couldn't stand. That great, angry, strange-coloured dog – the animal I couldn't contain – had gotten out of its crate again and now there were helicopters circling the farm.

Next to the Redbourn house, a guy called Timothy Gear lived with his parents in a mobile home – we reckoned they were living there till they got planning permission for something more permanent, which was fine by me. The real problem was that the local lads thought it would be fun to nick cars in Hemel or Luton or wherever, race them on the adjacent M1 (which was less than a mile across the fields from our place), jump off at exit 9, then down along our dirt track to Rabbitfield Springs, a small area of woods in the shape of a triangle near the farmhouse. The kids would do donuts and spins in the fields until they got bored and burned the cars out in the woods. I wasn't having that – Aaron and Kaley were little, and I was afraid they'd get hurt one day.

Plus, it scared Elvis and Priscilla, and I really couldn't afford for them to fly off again.

I decided to spend a bit of money to fix the problem. I paid about fifteen hundred quid to have a five-bar gate installed across the dirt lane and I padlocked it. There were four keys: I kept one; I gave another to Bill, the guy we'd taken in; the third I gave to Timothy Gear's father who lived in the mobile home and the fourth went to the girl who looked after all my bigger animals. Now there was nowhere for the kids to race the cars, and peace returned to the farm.

That day – 11 November 1997 – the drinking had started early. As much as I loved the outdoors, I also loved drinking, and the two often went hand-in-hand for me. I'd started with a lunchtime glass or two of red and, as the afternoon had gone on, I'd kept up a fairly steady rate. The shooting done, I headed to the Bell and Shears to have a few before home.

It was always notable that when my car pulled up outside the Bell and Shears, by the time I'd locked up and walked inside, every pint glass was empty inside. I suppose it was a coincidence; in any case, as usual I stood everyone a pint, including Bill who was in the snug.

'Oy, Bill, what's up mate? Everything OK up home?' I said.

There was a pause. Not a good sign.

'Not really, boss,' Bill said.

'What?'

'Your "mate" next door, the son, has put a rope around the fence and ripped it all out with a tractor because he couldn't get through with the padlock on.'

This guy had obviously not communicated with his father – who had a key – and must have thought I'd padlocked it so he couldn't get through. Now, I'm not sure what colour I saw when I heard what he'd done, but it wasn't good – something like a red mixed with black or something. If I hadn't had the drink all day I might have seen sense, but this kid next door already thought he was a tough guy and now he'd gone too far.

It didn't take me long to get to the farm; all the way there I was thinking, 'bastard', and the rage had grown and had eaten into me. The lad must have heard my car squeal up because when he appeared at the door of his mobile home I didn't even wait for him to come out – I gave him one right through the window.

And then I really let him have it.

What I didn't know was that Bill had only given me half of the story. The father had put the fence back in place before I got home, knowing I'd be upset. If I'd walked another 50 feet, I'd have seen there was no problem and gone about my evening. But the dark forces had gotten me and I set about the bloke with a real fury.

On the walk from his trailer to the farmhouse, my first thought was, how am I going to explain this to Tans? How am I going to turn it around to my favour? I might have been in the right to be angry – this lad had no reason to rip out the gate except to be a dickhead – but now I had to face Tans. And I hated – hated – upsetting her. I could deal with repercussions, because I'd had a lifetime on the edge. But she deserved better than this.

Her reaction? She was just worried I'd overdone it with the neighbour. That says everything you need to know about her.

But before we could really get into it, we heard the helicopters and then the armed response arrived (they knew I had guns on the property). A voice through a loud hailer told me to come out of the farmhouse with my hands up, and to get on the ground.

A cadre of men with guns drawn even edged past the garage. If they'd opened it, they'd have seen 150 knackered Russian TVs with questionable parentage. I think they might have asked me why I had a garage filled with Argos TVs . . .

As it was, they made me turn around, take the cuffs and lie there. I asked one of the officers if I could give Tans a cuddle before I left. He ignored me, put me in the back of a car and took me to St Albans' nick.

At the nick, I was processed, placed in a cell and then the worst thing of all: they took away all my clothes and made me wear a white paper suit. I hadn't been dressed up for a fight – I was still wearing my Wellington boots and plus twos. It seemed like overkill to me, but the police said they needed to look at the blood on the boots – it was pheasant blood, at least that's what I thought – but they needed everything to 'do forensics'. They put everything in brown paper bags and sealed them . . .

Forensics?

As the door of the cell closed, I suddenly started shaking violently. Forensics meant one thing: I'd killed the guy. It was one of the most terrifying moments of my entire life. Every time an officer came to the cell through the night I asked if I'd killed him, but they said they couldn't tell me.

I thought of Tans at home, alone all night, listening to the owl and wondering if I'd ever make it back. I'd let her down again and that was a terrible, terrible feeling. Because Tans had saved my life, over and over and over. And this was how I repaid her. She had been my defender for so long – sure, she'd let me have it once the dust settled, but in the moment she would step up for me again and again. She must have seen something in me that was better, purer, than the guy who drank too much and punched people through plate-glass windows. In fact, she must have seen more in me than I saw in myself. And that's one of the reasons I loved her so much – she saw a better version of me than anyone else ever had. I knew what my reputation was: the guy who grabbed Gazza by the danglies; the guy who got booked after three seconds of a match, and sent off in 12 others; the guy who delivered that famous leveller to Steve McMahon in the F.A. Cup Final in 1988, just 14 minutes after he'd shaken Lady Di's gentle little hand; the guy who'd had too many fights when he'd been drinking.

Tans knew all that, but she didn't think it was all of me, or even the important part of me. She saw the innocent kid. I wish everyone could have someone like Tans in their life – someone who knows you and still loves you.

I still have no idea how to live without that. I really don't.

The guy I'd beaten up didn't die, not even close; but I had

made a mess of him. At the subsequent trial in St Albans, I was convicted of actual bodily harm and criminal damage. It was pretty obvious I was going down the steps, perhaps for as much as six months.

Once again, Tans had to face the consequences of what I'd done. She was terrified; we both were. The magistrates could have easily sent me away, but instead I got 100 hours of community service and a fine of £1,150 for what I did that night. (If they'd seen the TVs, it might well have been 200 hours.)

Tans got only heartache. I wish I could go back and change the years when I was in the drink. Without it, I was fine. With it, well, she worried that things were going to go wrong. She'd say, 'Vinnie, everything is going great,' but she'd say it with trepidation.

I'm glad she got me sober for the last six years. She deserved more than that, but at least she got the little boy back full-time, the kid before the pain kicked in, a pain that was softened by the drink.

But she loved me whatever I was. That was the thing. She just loved, and when she loved – be it her grandfather, her mum and dad, her brother, her daughter, her friends, or me, who deserved it the least sometimes – well, it was without boundaries, a love bigger than the sky.

We couldn't stay at Redbourn after the fight – it was ruined – so we bought a new place we called Highfield House, on Box Lane in Boxmoor, about ten miles away. I'd been driving past it one day and seen the sign; I called the estate agent who said I was welcome to go in and have a look around. Well, the owner was a smart lady – she had a chocolate fountain on the go and, as you stepped in the house, all you could smell was the lovely aroma of melting cocoa. Done. I put ten grand down immediately. I was a movie star, now – yeah, me and Lassie – and that's how things went. Chocolate fountain, check, boom, the place was ours. (Other things that they recommend when you're trying to sell a house are brewing coffee and baking bread, of course, but a chocolate fountain would take some beating.)

It was a huge white house, which I made even bigger with an extension, but it wasn't ideal. The place was on a main road, so people honked their horns and rang our security bell over and over.

We moved into the house on Box Lane the day I thought I might be going to prison. When I wasn't sent down, we celebrated hard in our new home, but the problems didn't end there.

We had brought Bill along, and his caravan. It was a nice caravan, but I'm not sure the neighbours were delighted, to be honest. Thanks to her huge capacity to love, Tans used to take Bill to his doctor's appointments – years of drinking had really taken its toll, so much so that he spent a fair amount of time at Harefield, which of course Tans knew all too well. But he found it too hard to follow the doctor's advice and he was spiralling downwards.

The final straw came on the night of the premiere of *Lock, Stock and Two Smoking Barrels*. At an early screening, Tans had turned to me on the train on the way home and had told me that it was going to be huge. She was always so proud of me. *Lock, Stock* was the first script I'd ever read. Tans and I would sit in bed at night as I learned my lines. She'd read the other parts and, accidentally, the stage directions, too, which was hilarious.

BIG CHRIS [me]: I have got something for ya. Well, for your boy, actually.
JD [as voiced by Tans]: Well, I suggest you speak to him, then.

But then Tans carried on . . .

TANS: They all look rather shocked. He is carrying their bag and he places it on the table, which increases the shock factor.

I'd look up confused, then realize what had happened.
'Tans, just read what he's saying.'
'Oh, I'm sorry, I'm sorry,' she'd say. Sometimes she'd throw the script on the bed. 'I'm useless at this . . .'
'No, you're not, babe, you're not! Come on, let's keep going.' It was the best time; we were so excited and she was my biggest supporter.

By the time the premiere came around, I knew that this was the start of my life as a movie star, and Tans and I and her friend Mandy had gone into London to celebrate. (To prove that I still had one foot in the football life, though,

I took Ray Harford and Iain Dowie to that premiere!) It had been a great night. And I realized then and there that this was my future. I felt at ease acting; I could do it, and I could do it well. The reviews were positive, and the laughs kept coming throughout the night.

But as ever with me, the good times were leavened by the bad.

It turned out that Bill had finally lost the plot while we were in London at the premiere. He'd been drinking heavily again and he thought it would be a good idea that night to come into our house, steal all of Tans' transplant medication, then drive off in Mandy's car – some beat-up old Renault. He crashed it and was arrested. We only knew about it when Maureen, who was babysitting Kaley, called us to tell us that she'd been woken up with a bright light in her eyes. Figuring she'd finally thrown the celestial seven, she'd been amazed to see that instead of the holy host and the choirs triumphant, what was standing there instead was a local copper. Not Jesus, or the Blessed Mother – just Officer Plod, holding a torch. We already thought the house was haunted – there were various tales of a former lady of the house skulking around and scaring the crap out of people – so you can imagine Maureen's reaction when this big lunk of a copper woke her up by shining a light in her eyes.

By the time we got home, we knew it was the end of Bill in our lives. We'd looked after him for four years but we could no longer trust him.

As the years went by, Tans, too, no longer felt safe at Box

Lane. After *Snatch*, and my first lead role, in *Mean Machine*, my fame was at its height and too many people were ringing the bell or trying to get autographs, while I just wanted to give Tans the most beautiful, wonderful life I could, and one that was as private as possible, given what she had to go through every year of it.

12

A DAY AND A LIFE AT HAREFIELD

Tans was so brave about her regular trips to Harefield, but the truth is they scared her so much. After the transplant, she had to be monitored regularly, as the doctors really didn't have a timetable for how long the heart might work. Remember, these were still the early days of transplants, so Tans was an important marker for the whole endeavour. Consequently, they had her back to Harefield regularly to check her progress, which was good for both sides: she got looked at closely and her case was then used for research (she was especially fascinating to doctors because she'd been so young and seemingly healthy before her first heart had collapsed).

Tans took medicine twice a day, morning and evening. It was often my job to make sure it was taken every night. Wherever we were in the world or what time we went to bed, it had to be taken. There was the ciclosporin and the Imuran for anti-rejection of the heart; there were water tablets. Even if we'd had a bunch of drinks, we had to remember; fortunately, after all those years there was a kind of mechanism in her head, so she knew she had to take them. But if she'd had one too many glasses of champagne – really, that was her only vice when it came to drinking – then it became my job: 50mg of this, 25 of that, something else of the other. Actually, it would scare me to death that Tans would miss something – it wouldn't have killed her, but the whole regimen would have been out of sync and that would have been dangerous.

The ciclosporin was used to mitigate the chance of rejection, but it's a tough drug, especially as it can lead to a greater chance of cancers (nowadays, anti-cancer drugs are added to the regime). In addition, her immune system was suppressed by the drugs she took, which meant she was more prone to infections. Also, her kidneys were badly affected; she had the gout and there were two bouts of cervical cancer that she had to face. She was so tough about it all, but it was so much for one person to take.

It was the semi-annual and annual trips to Harefield, though, that were the biggest stresses for Tans.

We went together to Harefield for her check-ups; often, they'd coincide with her birthday (and, therefore, Kaley's), so it could get stressful in early April as the Harefield trip approached. Tans was determined though to be just another patient – yes, she was married to someone famous, but she never made anything of that at Harefield, and neither did I. When she was there, she was Tanya Jones, transplant recipient, not Tanya Jones, wife of Vinnie Jones. In fact, she had hundreds of offers through the years to do modelling or interviews and she turned it all down – she was adamant that nothing she did would appear to be exploiting the fact that Harefield had saved her life; she didn't want anything to appear as though she was special. Tans was terrified of letting the doctors down. She knew what she'd been given was such a privilege and she would never use my fame, or our fame, to jump in front of one person.

The days at Harefield would start early in the morning. We'd line up with everyone else and wait our turn for Tans to have blood work done, a stress test and an angiogram. The walk to the operating theatre where they did the angiograms was always terrifying to her. In the beginning, it could take a couple of days to get all the tests done, though later Tans could be in and out in a day. Still, she'd get herself all teary and scared on the way to the theatre and she'd make me promise that I'd be outside when she come out, which I was – every time. Tans always used to say to Dr Mitchell, 'Can I have a little bit more gin and tonic?' meaning the sedative. It was an incredibly invasive procedure – they'd have to send a little camera up through her groin and into the heart to check it was in good shape – but it was also stressful because we were afraid of what they might find. And Tans always said she could feel the camera going through her, which she found petrifying.

After the angiogram was complete, they'd wheel her into the recovery room and she'd have her little sleep. I'd have her little list of food to get for her because she'd be starving when she woke up. I would wait until she was comfortable, we'd do the kiss throw and catch thing as we always did when I was away somewhere, and then I'd fly up into the

155

town of Harefield to the bakers and get her stuff; she loved little cucumber sandwiches and cakes and crisps. As Tans came too, she saw all that food waiting for her and it was like Christmas morning for her.

Then, we waited. This was the hardest part. 'What do you think?' she'd say, over and over. 'What did Dr Mitchell say?'

I'd say, 'Oh, he's so pleased,' even though I hadn't spoken to him. Sometimes it would be 7 o'clock or 8 o'clock at night – the hospital became kind of spooky then – and we'd sit there holding hands, waiting for those results.

Eventually we'd troop down to Mitchell's office, and every time he'd say, 'Brilliant, Tanya! Heart's great.'

We lived off that. For weeks and months, we'd live on that because, in a real way, it was Tanya getting her life back all over again. At the start it was twice a year, then once, then every other year, but it was always the same: we'd stress and worry and fret that her heart had something wrong, and then they'd do the day of tests and we'd get the all-clear, and the sense of relief was so profound.

Going to Harefield really put things in perspective. Each time we'd try to avoid looking at the list that was up of recipients who were still alive, because we knew a lot of them. But that list got thinner and thinner as the years went by. One year, Tans asked a nurse about a guy called Tommy Flanagan – he was a lovely bloke she'd gotten to know over her time going back to Harefield. 'How's Tommy? Has Tommy been in?' Tans said.

There was a horrible pause and the nurse looked away. We knew what that meant. Tans used to get kind of angry because it would be all these names and written next to each one was, 'one year', 'two years', '10 years', '15 years', '20 years', but that list, with her on it, just got thinner and shorter.

There were other stresses at Harefield, too. People quite naturally wanted to talk to us – Tans was quite a famous recipient and I was well-known, too – but we just wanted to get our heads down, get on with it and get out. Tans shunned any limelight.

One day, I left her to go and get the food and when I got back, there was a woman I hadn't seen before in the room with her. Tans was recovering, still mostly out of it, and I asked the nurses who this woman was. They told me she'd claimed to be family, but certainly no one I'd ever heard of.

Let's just say that when it became clear it was a journalist pretending to be a friend of Tans, it didn't end that well for them.

To her dying day, Harefield was everything to Tans. She adored the staff – Dr Mitchell and the nurses. They were like angels to her.

With all the stress of having to go to Harefield regularly, and the bad publicity that I sometimes still got for my on-the-field antics, we needed somewhere much more private than Box Lane, so it was time to move again. This time, we picked a place in Tring, called Cedars.

This was a proper house – the dream house of our lives –

9,000 square feet on six acres. It was Charlie big bananas. You could get into third gear along the driveway, that's how long it was. We paid a million quid for it, then renovated it to the tune of another million.

We had six bedrooms, including the master suite that was the size of some houses. It was so big you could make a phone call across it. Kaley's room was vast, too – the best in the house, probably. The kitchen was 62 feet long by 30 feet wide, amazing. The house itself had an odd layout, though – it was sort of separated in the middle by a long walkway, open to the elements. I wanted to join it up properly, to make one structure of the whole thing, so I had huge arched windows built to fill the open spaces in the walkway. I even built a trout lake with a lovely fishing hut on it – a one-bedroom fishing hut! We had beautiful big avenues and lawns.

With my football career over, the movies had kicked in big time, as had other things in the world of entertainment.

In 2001, I somehow landed a gig appearing before the Queen in the seventy-third Royal Variety Performance. I sang and danced my way through 'Macavity the Mystery Cat' in a tribute to Andrew Lloyd Webber.

Before the show I found myself in a dressing room downstairs with Stephen Fry and Rowan Atkinson, until someone said, 'Oh, Elton's upstairs,' so I went up to see him instead. There was a ton of red wine there and Elton wasn't drinking, so I helped myself rather liberally – perhaps that's why, when I got to meet the Queen, I tipsily said, 'Is anybody using your Cup Final tickets this year, Ma'am?'

(This was November, so god knows why I thought she'd have her tickets already!).

Everyone told Tans she should meet the Queen too, but as ever she was just too modest and too supportive of me to care – 'This is Vin's night,' she said. Later, though, we convinced her to meet Her Maj, but instead of the usual 'Ma'am' rubbish, Tans just said, 'Oh, hello!' to her. We loved Tans for that; that was Tans – no bull, no side, just a real person.

A year later, on 2 November 2002, I was lucky enough to release a record called *Respect*. I'd always loved music, so this was a thrill for me. I covered a load of great songs – 'Everybody Needs Somebody', 'Dance to the Music', 'Dock of the Bay', 'High Ho Silver Lining', 'Mustang Sally', 'Gimme Some Lovin'', 'In The Midnight Hour' – and a whole bunch of others. I even got on *Top of the Pops* singing Jim Croce's 'Bad, Bad, Leroy Brown', which to my 15-year old daughter was pretty cool – if you look closely at the video of it, you can see her dancing away in the front row – a bit like her mum always being her brother's biggest supporter.

Tans supported her daughter completely, too.

Even when her health was out of whack, she'd show up at the lacrosse matches and the netball, at the sports day, or the plays, or at the cathedral when Kaley was in the choir. But Kaley was having a tough time at school. We'd sent her to Stowe – I always wanted the best education for my kids (we also sent Aaron to private school) – but the place was filled with kids who cared more about status than anything. They called her Mini Vinnie, which was ridiculous, and the day she accidentally caught someone in the face with a lacrosse stick of course the press had a field day given her connection to me. But it was a party at our new house that really brought it all to a head.

I was away filming *Eurotrip* and Kaley took the opportunity to invite some school friends over for a low-key party. Tans and her best friend at the time, Denise, were going to be there in the kitchen so nothing could go wrong. Kaley invited maybe 50 people, tops, but everyone in the whole school found out and they showed up. It was Easter break and they'd all travelled in from all over the country; it was ridiculous. They even brought tents with them. One boy proudly made it his business to go to house parties and trash the place – that was his thing, apparently. I wish I'd been there to see him.

The party quickly ran out of control and Kaley locked herself in our bedroom. Meanwhile, the kids discovered my stash of 100 bottles of 1985 Lynch-Bages – Tans caught one of them smashing a bottle open so that he could drink it.

It was a complete nightmare and made worse by the fact that one of the boy's dads worked for the *Daily Mail*. One boy had brought weed and he was smoking it in one of the bushes out front, so the *Mail* said it had been a druggy party, which it wasn't.

But it was a disaster – one kid even found Aaron's air rifle and blasted out the window in his room with it. Tans and Denise finally managed to get rid of everyone and called a glazier to fix the window. It was decided that the story would be downplayed for me; problem was, I found out about it via a little piece in the *Daily Mail*. Tans and Kaley didn't tell me about the window, though, so imagine my confusion a while later when I told Tans that I'd met a bloke who claimed he'd been at our house fixing a window – he even said that it had been shot out. I just thought the guy was high or something.

That party was the final straw for Kaley – she left Stowe after that and I don't blame her. And I also don't blame her and Tans for not telling me about it (though I should have guessed when I saw that our white carpets were no longer white).

They always had such a special bond, those two. There are lots of reasons for their closeness – daughters and mothers and all that for a start. But in their case, there was also the fact of how Kaley came into the world. She understood what her mother had gone through to give birth to her and Tans, in her turn, knew how near she'd been to never seeing Kaley grow up. Consequently, they were closer than anything; you really had to see it to believe it. This continued right up to Tans' dying day and, in the last year, I could see how Kaley's love became deeper and deeper, if such a thing was even possible, as she nursed her mother through the final stages of her illness.

I'm so proud of what Kaley did, and of who she is. She's one of the loveliest people you could wish to meet and she's been the rock that has held us all together. She's truly her mother's daughter, that much is for certain.

13

VIRGIN TO JAPAN

In May 2003, I took a flight to Japan. And everything came crashing down for *me* this time.

I wish drink wasn't even a part of this book; now, six years sober and counting, it feels like a different life. But I have to own what I did, and what happened on the Virgin flight to Japan was perhaps my lowest point. There's no excuse for it.

I had been drinking, as ever, and three hours into the flight I was chatting with some folks from Carlton TV at the bar of the aircraft in first class. I'd had too much; I got lairy at a guy who was trying to calm me down and I slapped him and pushed his head into a window. Then it got even worse: I went off at the guy again.

Eventually I fell asleep, but by the time I woke up in Japan, everything had changed in my life. As I told the press outside the court back in the UK in a statement, 'I regret the incident deeply and pleaded guilty to both counts. [I] will complete the punishment with grace and thank the court and the Probation Service.' And I meant it; what I did was boorish and awful.

It was only me who kept fucking it up, being a fucking stupid fucking bloke who wanted to be a fucking main show man, fucking boozing and taking his fucking childhood out on anybody that got in his way. In some ways these were wasted years – wasted years of love, in a sense.

There could have been more time and effort from me. But when I fucked up with the booze it was only Tans I was bothered about – hurting her was what killed me, punished me. Seeing her so desperately upset and what I'd done to her was my punishment.

I never told Tans this, but the night before sentencing, my lawyer for the air rage case told me, 'If we'd have gone to Crown Court, you'd have got nine months. As it's just the Magistrate's, you'll get three, and you'll do about six weeks. Bring your wash bag.' (I did indeed take a bag of toiletries to the court.) I got lucky in the end – I was probably the last person who ever had air rage like that and didn't go to prison. I got more community service and more fines, but I also suffered in bigger ways.

When the story broke, we hadn't been in the house in Tring all that long, and financially it was straining us as we'd gone over budget on the renovations. Knowing all that, my manager called Tans and gave her the truth: 'Tanya, get out. The dream's over. There's no repairing this. Sell that fucking house. Straight away. You've got to think of you. I'll look after Vinnie. There isn't much we can do. All the endorsements are going to end. You've got to sell that house and look after you and Kaley.'

It was tough to hear that he'd made that call, but he was right. I did indeed lose all my endorsements, everything. And I rated him highly for caring for Tans and Kaley that day. His name was Peter Burrell. He still looks after Frankie Dettori.

But I only tell this story so that you can know what Tanya Jones said when I got back from Japan.

At the airport on my return I was arrested, then charged. I couldn't believe that yet again I'd dropped Tans and Kaley into this kind of thing. When would I learn? I was so afraid of how hurt Tans would be; we'd finally gotten our dream house, spent all that money on it, and now this.

When I got out of jail, I drove home to her and Kaley. I was petrified – not for me, but for the hurt I'd caused her, and the fact that we were facing financial ruin.

And do you know what she said to me?

'I don't care about the house. I don't need six acres. Rent it out. Get us a caravan – you, me, and Kaley, in a caravan. I'm fine.'

How do you measure a life like the one Tanya Jones led? I'm trying to here, in these pages, but nothing I say will come close to the full worth of her. She wasn't a saint, or perfect, or too sweet to be true, or holier than thou. Tans was just the embodiment of love, of understanding, of caring for people. She fed Bill the homeless guy and took him to the doctor; she would spend hours listening to my friends open their hearts to her; she forgave all of us for our fuck-ups. If you were in with Tanya Jones, then you were in for life. She never forgot a slight – she was no pushover.

But if she loved you, she found a way to forgive you quickly and love you harder than ever before. Perhaps, because of what she went through giving birth to Kaley, she'd seen how life can be taken away and how precious it is, and how we should all make the most of every second. Sure, we fought sometimes, and she had that annoying habit of being able to remember everything from the night before, and from years ago, when perhaps you had had too much to drink and could barely recall anything. She wasn't about to waste time holding grudges, though.

So, I'd screwed everything on a Virgin flight and now I had to work out what to do. First thing was I rented the Tring house to Walter Swinburn, the jockey. I was afraid it would be way too big for him – he was a jockey, after all – but he had six kids, so he was all set. Then I did a few acting jobs and got a bunch of money together, enough to buy another place up the road on Shootersway, Berkhamstead. It was a great brick house, Georgian, imposing, big pillars outside – really beautiful. That was another dream I ticked off, living on Shootersway – when I was a kid, everyone knew Shootersway. You'd made it if you moved there. And I had, though in odd circumstances.

But already my life was half in the States and half in the UK. America was calling and I was falling for the place.

14

THE ZEBRA ON MULHOLLAND DRIVE

One day we were out shopping for stuff for our new house on Mulholland Drive, right next door to Quentin Tarantino. In the Galerie Michael on Rodeo Drive we found a zebra. Not a real one, mind, but a huge impressionistic painting of one. You had to look a few times to make out the face, but it was a zebra alright, and Tans and I clocked it at exactly the same time.

I said, 'We'll have that, shall we?'

Tans said, 'Yeah, we'll have that.'

This was our American adventure just beginning.

We'd rented a place to begin with and kept a foot in the UK by hanging on to the house in Shootersway because we weren't sure that we'd move to the States permanently. But then all that changed when I bought Tinker.

It was the day before Valentine's Day, 2007.

Tans and I were passing a pet store in Beverly Glen and we noticed a teacup Yorkshire terrier in the window, and I thought, 'Fucking hell, I've got to have that little puppy.' Tans was adamant that we were not getting a dog, so I pretended that she'd put me off, but I knew myself, and her, better than that. The morning of Valentine's Day I went back to the store and picked up the dog. I also bought a pine four-poster bed for it (I'd usually keep a dog in a cardboard box in the house, but this guy deserved better than that). Back at the apartment, I put the dog in the bed outside the door upstairs, banged on the door and ran back down to hide. Tans opened the door, screamed and shouted, 'Oh my god!' and that was it. Tinker, boom, done.

You'd think Tans had just given birth again – she loved that dog instantly. When she told Kaley about it, it was clear to Kaley that we were staying for good.

So this was it: this was L.A. life done big. We had bought the place on Mulholland for a million and a half and probably spent another million on it, all told. And the zebra was crucial.

It was the first thing we did, hanging that zebra. Then I had the two walls out front both painted with the word 'sunshine' for the John Denver song Tans loved so much, 'Sunshine on My Shoulders'. Then we did everything out to match the zebra theme: black-and-white throughout, with glass and chrome, that's all. Zebra-themed high chairs at the kitchen counter; zebra-print throw cushions on the cream couch; outside, a cabana for the men with a black-and-white Union Flag on the wall and another cabana for the women. Deep brown covers on the beds, facing a black fireplace. I even hung a signed picture of Alan Shearer wearing his black-and-white striped Newcastle kit in the gym. Sure, there were flashes of colour: my big red Sex Pistols poster; photos of Tans looking as gorgeous as ever; a poster for *Snatch*, just off the living area. But even the poster for *X-Men: The Last Stand*, in which I played Juggernaut, was mostly black-and-white.

And we filled that house with people, including Kaley. Realizing we were staying for good, Kaley, who was 21, joined us, bringing her dog, a bichon frise called Baby. Sadly, Baby didn't do well after her long trip. She never seemed to settle and, after a couple of years, I found her dead in her little bed. Burying her that day loosed something very strong in me; I cried and cried and cried as I dug a place for her to rest in the backyard at Mulholland. Perhaps I realized that nothing lasts forever, even as we built an extraordinary new life in the United States.

We truly did create the most unbelievable Los Angeles life-style at 'Sunshine'. Non-stop friends arriving at the door; non-stop people coming in from England. We thought it might wear off, but it didn't – it just kept going.

For Tans' birthday each year I would fly Julie and Joanne, her two best friends, over for her. She never wanted a Gucci bag or a Louis Vuitton purse – no, she just wanted her two best friends. And it's no exaggeration to say that she got as excited the fifteenth time they came as the first time. She'd leave insanely early to pick them up from the airport. I'd say, 'Babe, it's an hour, hour and a half to the airport. Why are you leaving five hours before they land?' but there was no stopping her.

And still everyone kept coming. LAX airport became like

a revolving door for us, because as Tans was dropping people off, others would be arriving. In the first year of us living in the States, she did 62 separate trips to LAX – she'd literally drop people off at departures, kiss, hug, all that, then run up to arrivals to greet the next lot, more kisses, more hugs. Sometimes it was my sister's family, or her family, or all of mine. And then friends and more friends and more friends.

Tans was so happy, welcoming everyone, making sure they were settled, giving them tours of L.A. We nicknamed them Tans' Tours. She'd do them in my old Cadillac convertible – that car would be full of kids and friends and it was swaying around . . . Tans would drive everyone up to the Hollywood sign, then they'd drive around all the houses in Beverly Hills. She always made sure to stop at Priscilla Presley's house – she loved Priscilla. She probably saw something of herself in Elvis's wife – the woman married to the famous guy. Then they'd all head off to Venice and Santa Monica, where she'd get a henna tattoo, every time: it always said, 'I love Vin'.

With the henna in place, Tans would make sure she got her palm read. She and all the girls would head off to some spiritualist and fork over their 50 bucks or whatever; she loved all that. To end the day, she'd take everyone to the Hot Wings Cafe on Melrose, or Mel's Diner, or some deli up in Beverly Glen. Wherever she went she always wanted the chicken wings. She didn't like fancy places where the Hollywood women would go to be seen and do lunch. She wanted to be with her family and friends and eat chicken wings. Sometimes potato skins, but usually wings.

And it would take all day because of Tans' driving.

Tanya Jones was the only human being who ever drove around Los Angeles without using the freeway. You really have to know what L.A. is like to appreciate what that means. L.A. is basically one big freeway, or a whole load of big freeways. There's the 5 and the 10 and the 101 and the 110 and the 210 and the 405 and the 605 and the 710 and on and on and on. Los Angeles is very spread out, too – to get a sense of scale, it's about 45 miles from San Fernando in the north to Long Beach in the south; that's basically Watford to Sevenoaks as the crow flies.

So, to get around you will definitely have to use a freeway or several . . . and everyone talks about how they got somewhere and what freeway they used. There's a really funny skit on *Saturday Night Live* called 'The Californians' where all they do is compare freeway routes and that's what it's like there. (One of my favourite bits in 'The Californians' is when Fred Armisen shouts at Bill Hader, 'Get back on San Vincente, take it to the 10, then switch over to the 405 north, and let it dump you out at Mulholland where you belong!')

None of this mattered to Tans, though – she never used the freeways. And she drove everywhere at 22 m.p.h.

One year, my son Aaron came to stay and, being a military lad, he had an idea to see the RMS *Queen Mary*, a legendary cruise ship/troop carrier which is docked in Long Beach, right at the bottom of L.A. – it's basically as far south as you can go before you fall into the Pacific Ocean. 7475 Mullholland is about 40 miles to the north and, at rush hour, in the worst traffic, it takes about an hour and a half to get down there (you can take the 101 to the 710, or jump on the 5 in Glendale and pick up the 710 in East L.A. – see? Everyone talks about which freeway to use, even me.)

Everyone, as said, except Tanya Jones. She quite happily offered to drive Aaron to see the *Queen Mary*, but she had no intention of taking the 5, the 101, the 710 or any freeway, in fact. No, she was going to stick to local roads and, like Mr Magoo, she was going to peer over the steering wheel and stick to her 22 m.p.h.

Tans and Aaron left at 10 a.m. . . . . and arrived just before 6 p.m. I think the *Queen Mary* was closed, actually, so they drove right back. I was well asleep when they finally made it to the house.

Aaron had had a wonderful day, nonetheless. That was Tans. Life and soul. Best person ever.

Tans driving was the funniest thing, because it didn't matter whether the car had cost a hundred grand or five dollars – she was in a world of her own. Driving with her was a nightmare, to be honest, but it was even worse having her as a passenger. She'd shout, 'You're going too fast! You're too close! That lane! That lane!' Fortunately, she was quite happy to ride in the back – anything to avoid the front with me, and I wasn't going to argue; she was a terrible passenger. She just couldn't get over someone else – i.e., me – driving a bit faster than her 22 m.p.h.

Not only that, but when she drove, she was completely oblivious to everything around her. She'd say, 'Oh, why do they keep beeping at me?' Most days she'd come home and

172

say, 'Oh, this bloke was really going mad and waving his fist at me. And I was just driving along . . .' She just didn't get it, the driving part. It was so funny.

When we lived next door to each other at Hunter's Oak, Tans was driving a real old banger, an old black Citroën, with stuff hanging off it. Suzy Barnes, who was married to John Barnes at the time, lived up the road, and they had the superstar lifestyle – the red Mercedes, the whole bit. Suzy would beg Tans to not embarrass her. 'Tans, please,' Suzy would say, 'don't park outside the house with that car.'

Tans was having none of it.

'Shut up, Suzy,' Tans would say, 'it gets me from there to there!' But god knows how – the thing didn't have a lick of oil in it. I tried to drive it one day and it sounded terrible – when I popped the bonnet, it was as dry as a bone. So, on our first Valentine's Day together, I bought her a car – a little black Mazda sportscar with a personalized number plate: 20 TJ. (She *hated* that plate; she was so modest, always. I've always loved plates; I've had loads, and I've bought them for her mum and for Kaley, but Tans never cared for them.)

Even though she was a terrible driver, she still had taste – and Tans' dream car was a red Bentley. I bought her one of those in the end, too. She had it about four years, but then she was too sick to drive it.

But money was never the point for Tans. From the day we stayed up all night talking in Hunter's Oak to the night she died, she didn't know to the nearest £10, £100, or hundred grand how much we had in the bank. She never saw a statement; she never asked to see a statement. All her stuff, all her jewellery, Cartier, Louis Vuitton – I bought all of it. She never once came home with a Louis Vuitton bag, never once said, 'I bought myself some new shoes.' Everything she bought would be from H&M or Venice Beach. She'd say, 'I bought two dresses for 40 dollars!' She looked better than anyone, but she'd be in a $20 dress – it looked like a $20,000 dress on her. Tans always looked a million times better than anyone – she was gorgeous and gracious and she didn't have a hundred grand dripping off her arms and ears. Tans didn't even have her ears pierced. She'd go to Cartier and buy me a lighter or something for my birthday and buy herself nothing.

So, cars? It honestly didn't matter to her whether she was driving a little Citroën or a 150-grand Bentley. And it wouldn't matter to me either, if she was still here to drive at 22 m.p.h. What I'd do to see that again.

We were living the grand L.A. lifestyle, but I hadn't even been sure I wanted to move there initially.

I had done a movie called *Gone in 60 Seconds* – the first one – and everybody was telling me I needed to move to L.A. if I wanted to be a big star. During filming I was really missing Tans, who'd stayed back with Kaley who was still in school. It was 2 a.m. and it was really hot in downtown L.A. I called her and said, 'It's fantastic here. Babe, I'm walking around missing you, but it's two in the morning and it's boiling hot.'

And that was it. Tans said, 'OK, yeah. We're coming. We're going to come.' And they did.

We had a wonderful, wonderful, ridiculous time at that Mulholland house. We were up there next to Tarantino, for a start; tour buses would swing by every five minutes. I had a Union Flag flying proudly over the property. There were huge electric gates next to the signs reading 'Sunshine' and, once inside, Tans was so proud to show everyone how I'd remodelled and rebuilt the place around the zebra theme. I was making movies, and tons of dough, and I managed the Hollywood All-Stars football team, too.

We had some amazing people on that team: Dermot Mulroney, Jason Statham, Ziggy Marley, Robbie Williams, Eric Wynalda, John Harkes and Frank Leboeuf, to name just a few. And I took it seriously. Forget John Sitton ranting at his Leyton Orient players and his famous, 'And you can bring your fucking dinner 'cos by the time I've finished with you, you'll fucking need it.' Forget Neil Warnock's infamous rant at his Huddersfield Town players ('Third in the league, and we've got two thousand fans getting pissed on!'). Forget Phil Brown making his Hull players sit on the pitch at Manchester City at half time – here's a partial transcript of one of my half-time team talks to Hollywood All-Stars:

What I do get pissed off with is the fucking decisions. When there's a guy stood in front of you there, why go for this fucking worldy, when it is 90 degrees?

Danny, you're six-three and you ain't won a fucking header all day. I've been in the game too long, Danny,

175

for this bollocks. Either fucking win it or fucking get off.

We've got to do the fucking hard work. John and Ollie, your job is in the middle of midfield. You can't be going fucking roaring in like fucking Roy of the Rovers. It's too fucking hard.

Don't waste my fucking time on a Sunday by coming here and wanking it off. This is just fucking bullshit. That looks to me like some of you have had a game this morning, some of you have got fucking airports on your mind. We're here for an hour and a fucking half, let's worry about this, not who you're picking up from airports. The effort here is dog shit.

Mikey – fucking get in there or I'll fucking throw a chair on for you. Will you be more comfortable then, if you're sitting down?

I'm fucking gutted for the lads on the fucking sideline, because they shouldn't be fucking there. All the fucking time and effort that goes into this fucking club. Lads, I've been at the highest level you can get, I can see who's fucking cheating. I can see that nearly run. Danny, I can see all that, 'Oh, the sun's in my eyes.' It ain't in his eyes, is it?

I'm telling you something right now – my money's on them winning this game unless you can show me one bit of fucking character. There's my prediction: my money's on them, unless you wankers can fucking pull yourself out the fucking bed and fucking get in here, and fucking work hard, and win the fucking ball.

Get yourselves sorted out.

Shakespeare eat yer heart out.

The Hollywood All-Stars games were on a Sunday, which was fantastic because we turned it into a proper day out.

All the girls used to get ready, Tanya and all her mates, to come down to watch. There was a little outdoor restaurant right on the side of the football pitch and Tans would arrive and be the anchor of it all; she was a fantastic entertainer.

The few times Tans *didn't* come down to football, I'd call her and say, 'All the lads are going to come back. We're on our way, would you go get 40 steaks?' By the time we'd get back she would have phoned a couple of her mates and they'd be there too; there'd be steaks going on the barbecue, the full Monty. And the house was spotless and there'd be food and drink, as much as you want. It was one of the highlights of our lives together – us lads in one cabana, eating steaks under a black-and-white Union flag; Tans and her girlfriends in the other cabana, having a few drinks and probably comparing horror stories of us lads. Most Saturday nights too there would be 30, 40 people at our house. We had the off license on speed dial.

But then the first signs of Tans' cancer arrived. Weirdly, if you say 'skin cancer' it doesn't sound as bad as some of the other kinds, and I think that's how we viewed it, at least initially. Kaley remembers that she was getting something out of the fridge in the house on Mulholland when her mum offhandedly told her that they'd found a bit of cancer, but it was nothing to worry about. 'I have really good doctors, they found it early, they can treat it, nothing to lose sleep over, darling,' Tans said. Kaley remembers being comforted by that. Like all of us, she figured her mother had been through worse and prevailed.

We never thought it would lead where it led, and we stayed hopeful, but it felt like we needed a new kind of lifestyle in any case. I gave up the team and we had to put a line under those years. It was time to sell Mulholland. I instigated the decision (well, me and the termites we found).

It was time to change everything once again. We were never really the full-on Hollywood types in any case and now we wanted to build ourselves something away from the hype. So, in the meantime, while we searched for the perfect place, we rented a place on Greenleaf Street in North Hollywood, about 15 minutes west of Mulholland.

Even though we loved all our friends and family, and had a brilliant time getting them all together, we were at our best watching a film on the couch in our sweats or pyjamas – that was better than any premiere. It just wasn't us. We surprised a lot of people, I think, by never being the couple who were open to this premiere or that party. We weren't that couple at all; it didn't really interest her. For us to be home having a cuddle on the sofa, making dinner, and then watching a film or something, that's what we wanted. Tans didn't want to be out in Hollywood with people who are not interesting or kind or real. And she was completely unfazed by stardom – she once told a story to *OK!* magazine about me being an actor: 'It's not such a big thing. People say things like, "Wow, how was it with Madonna," and I just reply, "Yes, she was ever so nice."'

That was Tans to a tee.

15

SOUTH DAKOTA

People loved Tanya Jones – everyone used to say, 'I love Tans; I just love her.' And it was genuine, every time.

Tans would listen to you – but I mean really listen to you. It was never about her. She wouldn't say, 'Now look, I've had a heart transplant and I did this and that and you should do this and you should do that.' Never. Instead, it was always about what the other person needed, who they were, how they felt.

There's a guy called Eamon O'Connor, a younger friend of Tans' dad – he's actually about my age – who everyone calls Archie. He and Tans had an incredible bond. She loved him because he'd been an underdog in his life, though he'd made good, and she loved an underdog. He loved her like everyone did and for the same reasons: because she was genuine, and kind, and warm, and would listen to you – really listen.

Archie came over to the States to play in a golf tournament one year and one night, as everyone was going to bed, Tans said to me, 'I'm just going to stay up and have a chat with Archie.' She came to bed pretty late that night and the next day I asked her how her chat had gone. Tans said that Archie had opened up to her about his life. People did that with Tans, they just unconditionally opened up to her. She was an angel to a lot of people. In fact – and this is no word of a lie – people thought she was an actual fucking angel.

There were too many times when Tans had to be an angel to me when I didn't deserve it.

Recently, I spoke to a psychologist, and he asked me, 'When were you at your best? When did you feel you were a nice guy, when you didn't want to fight, had no anger issues, didn't jeopardize everything positive in your life?'

My answer was this: 'Up to when I was 16, 17, 18, something like that.'

The psychologist said, 'And what happened to you at 16, 17, 18?' And the penny dropped. He said, 'That's when you started drinking alcohol, isn't it?'

Thank god Tanya knew me before the alcohol. I think that's what ultimately saved us after things like the air rage, the neighbour. She knew the true me. I went through a lot as a kid, and she understood that. It wasn't an excuse. It wasn't as if I'd say, 'Oh, it's the fucking breakup of that, and it's my dad and it's my mum, and it's the this and it's the that.' But she did understand it. She was the best reader of my soul.

Now it was up to me to find the good me, which involves no alcohol.

In 'Where Do You Go to My Lovely', our favourite song, there's a line that goes, 'Two children begging in rags / Both touched with a burning ambition / To shake off their lowly-born tags', and when I hear those words I feel the song was written for us. For me to buy that little girl a red Bentley on her fiftieth birthday, us driving out the showroom with it ... well, we couldn't contemplate how fully our lives had changed. We used to go into hotels – I remember one in Mauritius in particular that was ridiculous – and we'd be shown to the best suite. But the minute the door closed, we'd jump up and down in glee, like we'd gotten away with something. We were still the council house kids.

For 27 years together we were a fantastic social couple, but all I was doing was showing her off to everyone. I look at the photos of her now and I can't believe I was hers for all those years.

There's one photograph in particular I adore. We were attending Matthew Vaughn and Claudia Schiffer's wedding in May 2002. In the photo, she's wearing this amazing pink dress, high heels and swinging a little pink handbag. She's saying something to the camera, smiling, and I know what she was saying.

'Oh yeah, yeah, yeah. We do this every Saturday, Claudia Schiffer's wedding . . .' That's what she was saying to me; we were in on the joke together. Just like when she described Madonna as 'ever so nice'. Nothing got to her. She never got too big for herself. And for some reason, she chose me.

Tans chose me.

I wish I could just remember Tans as she was in that photo at Matthew and Claudia's wedding – smiling, confident, hopeful, healthy. But time was cruel to her, as it was to all of us. It's true that in 1987, when her heart collapsed, everyone around her would have taken just one more day, one more week, one more month, maybe one more year – they'd have taken anything just to have her alive for a little while longer. What god granted the Lamont family, what god granted all of us, was more than three decades, which is a true miracle. What you want, though, is eternity with someone like Tans. When you're given an angel, how do you let that angel go back to heaven? Well, let me tell you, you can't.

Tans struggled with health issues every day after the transplant. She got used to it: the kidney problems, the gout, the cervical cancer, the seizures, swallowing her tongue, a blood clot on her lung. Tans fought all of it with such incredible grace; she was the strongest person you ever met. She never complained; she just felt she'd been given a gift by Dr Yacoub and Dr Mitchell and everyone at Harefield. By the German boy whose heart beat in her chest, strong and true, every day. Yes, she had to take medicines twice a day, every day; yes, she had to suffer through the fear of what the follow-up visits to Harefield might reveal; yes, the angiograms were invasive and upsetting. But you'd never get a peep out of her about any of it. Tans was built of strong stuff and I think that's why we thought she'd outlast all of us. That's one of the reasons that losing her has been so hard. Tans would get beaten down and she'd bounce right back up. It happened every single time, so when she had some skin cancer scares, we thought she'd beat it like she always had.

But it was not to be. What saved her life ultimately took her life. How do you weigh the pros and cons of that? You can't. You just do what she did: you get up every day, you make the bed and you face forwards, hopeful and sunny, at a world that has no opinion about you.

The drugs Tans took to avoid her heart being rejected by her body also lowered her immune system and, crucially, they upped her chances of getting certain forms of cancer. One of those elevated risks was for skin cancer. After 20 years of taking those drugs, the odds get shorter and shorter that something bad is going to happen. And it did.

Tans was vigilant about having her skin checked out; she knew the risks and lived with them, but wasn't blasé about it. For the last decade of Tans' life, it felt like we were at the dermatologist on a monthly basis. I had a scare with the skin cancer too, but for Tans it was much more dangerous, given her medical history. On every visit, her doctors would inspect every inch of her body, checking every little mole or blemish. They would freeze them and cut them out.

Living in L.A., the risks were greater for skin cancer, obviously – certainly more dangerous than living in the UK. The trade-off was that she was less likely to be prone to infections, given that we lived in a much warmer, less damp environment. Of course, we had grown up in the UK back when fears about skin cancer were less prevalent; we just didn't really consider it, given that the sun seemed to shine twice a year at most. I think a lot of people of our generation were not even remotely clued in about the risks; some of us are paying for it now, of course. Tans always wore a hat in L.A. and was religious about using sunscreen, but it was still there in the back of our minds that we had to be vigilant about it. Who knows if the sun in the UK or the sun in L.A. did the damage; we'll never know, and it doesn't matter now.

For a while, after we moved to the States, Tans would go back and forth regularly to Harefield to have her heart check-ups. Back then, pre-existing conditions weren't covered by health insurance in the States. But with the passing of Obamacare, that changed. We were always so thankful to Obama for that; it was just the humane thing to do, and it meant that Tans, for one, could now get treatment at an affordable rate in the States as well as at Harefield.

Harefield was where she felt safest, so she'd still travel back there for her angiograms, but at Cedars-Sinai, they were able to do her bloods and give her a stress test, all that. Not having to travel as much was a great help to Tans, and at Cedars she was treated as a medical celebrity, given that they didn't have people who had transplants who had survived for so long. By 2010 it has been 23 years, which is approaching some kind of record. Still that heart beat on, strong and sure, and the doctors at Cedars would come by to meet this rock star of a survivor. She remained completely modest about it; in fact, she didn't like the attention one bit. To her, what had happened in 1987 was a miracle that she wasn't about to ruin by being all big-headed about it. Life was precious – she'd learned that and she cherished what Dr Yacoub had given her.

Even though she liked to shun the limelight, Tans encouraged me to do new stuff. In 2010 she convinced me to do series 7 of *Big Brother*. When it came to things like that, we all discussed it – me, Tans, Kaley, whoever it would affect. I really didn't want to do *Big Brother*, but Tans wanted people to see the real me, not the tabloid monster I was sometimes painted as. I guess it worked out in the end; I was there for a month, right up to the last day, and came third.

Before I went in, I promised Tans I wouldn't drink; god only knows how it would have gone if I hadn't avoided the booze in that situation. It was hard to leave her for so long. As ever, on the day I was leaving, she said, 'Where's my kiss?' and I threw her one to catch.

Once inside the *Big Brother* studio, I just did my own thing. Mostly, I cleaned. I'm very OCD, so I was cleaning everything, bleaching everything. Meanwhile, Tans and her mum were sitting up in bed at the Grove Hotel in Hertfordshire, eating room service and watching the show.

What people didn't know was I'd gotten to Davina McCall right before we started. She'd noticed that I was really apprehensive, and so I just asked her one thing: 'You don't know what's going to come out while you're in there, do you? People slaughter you. Will you do me a favour? When I come out the door evicted, give me the thumbs up if everything's cool, or a thumbs down if the shit's hit the fan, so I can prepare myself before the press get to me.' So, when I got evicted right on the last day and came out, I looked at Davina and she gave me the thumbs up. And then I was buzzing.

The whole thing had been insanity – people had dressed up like farm animals, Davina had dressed up like a chicken and I'd had to make up the fact that I'd been a cross dresser. (I can't tell if that's better or worse than dressing like a chicken to be honest.) But I'd survived one more ordeal.

I was still able to make Tans lose sleep over things, even when it wasn't my fault. When I was drinking, I think she was always worried what the fucking phone call would be. And it was also true that if everything was going brilliantly, she would often say, 'Oh no, no, everything's going too well – something bad is going to happen.' And this time, something bad did happen; but for once, it wasn't down to me.

A couple of years before *Big Brother*, on the first night of a hunting trip to Sioux Falls, South Dakota, in December 2008, I was attacked in a bar called Wileys in the centre of town. Some guys playing pool got in my face about this and that and then one of them went off and glassed me. It was a bad one; there was blood everywhere. As I went to clean myself up in the restroom, I was then approached by another guy, a friend of the first, and defended myself when it looked like he wanted to have a go too. The result was

I was charged with three counts of simple assault for the second fight; the first, in which I was glassed, was eventually deemed 'mutual combat'.

The glassing was catastrophic. I had two large gashes on my forehead, my ear was dangling down and my nose was basically hanging off – in all, I had to have 68 stitches and it was only by a fluke that I hadn't been blinded. I was very worried that the scars might severely affect my chances to get acting work too; I know I mostly play hard guys, but I didn't want to look like the Elephant Man.

After I'd been stitched up and released from jail, I went back to the hunting lodge. It was in the middle of nowhere, a Bear Grylls kind of place, and no one from the outside world would ever know I was there. I had my story for Tans all planned; I decided to say nothing about the assault, so that I didn't scare her. I was going to just tell her that the Land Rover had gone off the road and crashed and I hit the windscreen. But bad news will catch up with you somehow, and always pretty quickly in my case. That night, I got a message to call my manager, right there in the middle of wild South Dakota, and my stomach just dropped. I knew it was out.

The way it got out was a tiny bit funny, actually. I'd been on a pheasant shoot, but TMZ, the gossip channel, got their wires crossed, and heard it that I'd 'shot a peasant'. So, they went digging, the bar sold them the footage of the altercation and Vinnie was yet again about to be slaughtered by the press, as well as by people who knew me.

It's lonely when that happens. Usually, I would raise my

hand and take responsibility for the stupid things I'd done, like the air rage incident, or the time I was larking around in Ireland, bit a journalist's nose in jest and got more headlines than the hooligans who'd forced the Ireland–England game to be abandoned that same night. And the attitude of the press was set in stone – when I'd got sent off against Georgia, one reporter wrote, 'It was the final, unsavoury act of the season for the Jones boy', as though 'the Jones boy' (I was 30 when it happened) was some kind of ill-bred servant from below stairs.

But in this case, in Sioux Falls, I'd been set upon and nearly blinded. Unfortunately, that meant people would weirdly gloat about it. Some would say, 'What's he done *again*?' Few people understood that the truth was that our lives were once again in turmoil. For good news – a new and exciting acting role or doing well on *Big Brother* or the *X-Factor* – the calls were scarce. But something like Sioux Falls happens, and the phone rings off the hook with, 'What's he been up to?' It's horrible. When there's no support, you feel hellish lonely. And as hard as it was on Tans, it was terrible on Kaley and Aaron.

We did everything we could to shield them from the bad press, but once in a while it was impossible. I remember Tans calling me screaming from her car that the paparazzi had shown up at Kaley's infant school because they knew they could find Tans there at pick-up time. Tans understood they might show up when she and I were out in public, but at Kaley's school? We were big enough to deal with it, but it's completely unfair on the kids and the rest of the family.

But whatever the morals of it all, the simple fact remained: Tans was going to find out what really happened in Sioux Falls and once again she'd be scared and upset. According to Kaley, she and her mum were at Norm's gas station on Sunset Boulevard at the foot of the Hollywood Hills. My manager called Tans, and I don't know what he said, but it was something that scared her so much that she threw the phone at Kaley. Kaley talked to him and then explained to Tans what was going on. By the time they got home, the videos of the assault had been posted and Tans watched them and knew straight away it wasn't my fault this time. She said to Kaley, 'Given his past record, it's harder for people to believe; people will read the headline before they watch the video, and that will be that. But this one wasn't him.'

I flew back to Burbank airport the next day and the second Tans saw me she burst into tears. The ride home was brutal; I was still in bandages and Tans was freaking out, but she supported me 100 per cent on this one. She knew that if I was in the wrong, I'd hold my hand up and say so; I didn't, because I wasn't in the wrong.

There were bigger forces at play, though, bigger than just an assault charge. At the time we were working on getting our citizenship and if I'd been convicted, it would have been curtains for us. My previous convictions in the UK had never resulted in jail time and were not considered crimes of 'moral turpitude', as the Americans call it, so they wouldn't necessarily count against us in our application. But this incident in South Dakota could be bad. If I was convicted of assault in this case, I faced little or no chance of getting citizenship and once again a dream would have been over.

As it was, after a one-day trial in May 2009, I was cleared of all the charges. This didn't stop my assailants suing me, of course. I paid one off to get rid of him, but the one who glassed me bolted before he even gave his deposition when he realized he didn't stand an earthly.

Back in Los Angeles and healing up, we had to face what Tans was going through with her cancer. And it was about to get much worse.

16

THE BLOW-UP HEART BALLOON

We'd kept the house at Hunter's Oak, Hemel Hempstead, and we'd also bought Tans' grandmother's house on Gander's Ash. One day, when Tans was doing it up, she'd been taking the vacuum cleaner upstairs when she thought she'd pulled something in her side. She was in a lot of pain.

We flew to Dubai not long after, and the pain was getting worse. It was unlike her to complain, but she was in so much discomfort – truly awful, awful pain. And the pain brought on some fears and doubts in Tans – she'd sometimes say, 'You won't leave me, will you, Vin?'

Tans had been treated for her skin cancer, and it seemed to have gone well, but when we got back from the Middle East, around April 2015, Tans went to have an X-ray and it turned out her ribs were cracked. Of course, the doctors asked her if she'd fallen, or had had an accident or something, but she couldn't think of anything. This is one of the brutal things about cancer: Tans had beaten the melanoma, or so we thought, but the cancer had then snuck back into a different place. Now it was her ribs – the tumours had made the bones so brittle that they'd cracked – and there were worrying shadows on her lungs too.

This was a terrible turning point. We were supposed to be going to La Quinta, our place in Palm Springs, for the weekend, when she got the phone call that the cancer was back. I remember she was crying – her hair had just grown back after the skin cancer treatment and now she knew she was going to lose it all again. And honestly, from that moment on, the battle would be pretty much a constant thing. We didn't know it at the time, but we were facing a long road, with a terrible destination.

For the rest of her life, I don't remember Tans not having some kind of treatment, whether it be chemo or radiation. Her mother would always fly over, and if she was coming for a while, and it wasn't Christmas, then it signalled that something was very wrong, and that Tans was very scared.

But to Kaley, and to others, Tans was strong. She'd tell her daughter that she was going to be OK, that she'd got through everything, and Kaley believed her because Tans always *had* been OK. In Kaley's mind, her mother had survived a heart transplant, so she could survive everything; Tans was going to live forever.

I think we all tell ourselves this kind of thing all the time. That's because the fires are too hot, too hard to look at straight on. How could we contemplate a world in which Tans wasn't there? We couldn't; no one could. She had saved all of us from a life without her and now our brains couldn't conceive of her not being there every day, making our worlds better. So, when she said she'd win, we truly believed her. Of course we did. She deserved nothing less.

But there were many times when she couldn't hide what she was going through. There were terrible side effects to do with the chemotherapy and she'd also have to take fentanyl – a powerful opioid painkiller – for the pain in her ribs. That drug in particular made her feel like she was losing her independence because she couldn't drive herself anywhere. Kaley was working full time during the day and I was often filming, so Tans and her mum would have to Uber to doctor's appointments. It got to the point where Kaley realized she couldn't let that happen anymore and it was a big turning point for her. Once Kaley saw it for herself, close up – the radiation place with all the other people there, and then the doctors explaining things and not trying to protect her as her mum had often done by playing things down . . . well, then it was truly devastating for Kaley.

Fortunately for Kaley, she'd found someone who was to help her, and all of us, through the next few years.

Kaley and Lauren had started as friends and their friendship had deepened until, one night, they'd had dinner together and then, when they got home, they'd sat together in our driveway listening to music. Lauren had played 'Coconut Skins' by Damien Rice and Jack White doing 'Jolene' and a whole bunch of songs by Fiona Apple, and Kaley realized she'd never heard this music before and loved it. Kaley came in eventually and was telling Tans all about Lauren and the music, and Tans just said, 'Oh my god, darling, you're in love.' It was just like the moment

Maureen had said the same about Tans and me all those years ago.

Kaley wasn't convinced, until a moment in 2016 – 19 August – when Tans was rushed to Cedars-Sinai with a bad infection. Kaley stepped out to call Lauren to tell her what was happening and Lauren said she'd be right there. When Kaley came back into the room, even though she was so sick, Tans said again, 'Something's happened, you're in love.'

This was about six months after Tans had first said it to Kaley but this time Kaley just said, 'Yes.' A little while later, as she'd promised she would, Lauren turned up, and she's never left to this day. I don't know how we'd have survived without Lauren, actually. Sometimes people come along for incredible, magical, unseen reasons. When they do, cling on to them as long as you have strength in your arms.

Tans started to have more 'poorly days' where she needed to rest. If Maureen was there, Tans would ask her to make her a bacon sandwich or something, and we'd all treat it like a rainy day in. After Tans had had the chemo, it was inevitable that she would need a couple of those 'poorly days' and then she would say, 'Right, I want to go down to La Quinta.' She loved it down there – we both did – and the sunshine raised her spirits.

This became our new normal – Tans would have chemo every other week and we knew she was going to be a bit poorly for few days afterwards and need to rest at home, and then she would be back at it, always planning something, always having someone come and visit her – Shane, or her friends Jo and Julie, or whoever it was. Tans was always planning something and always looking forward to something. She was the most positive person you could imagine, even in the face of all this pain and discomfort.

We really thought we'd beat it; truly, we did. Right up until Christmas Eve 2018. That's when I think we both knew. Yeah, we knew.

Tans had been complaining of headaches through the latter part of 2018. Given that she was so susceptible to cancer – she was still having treatment for her ribs and her lungs – and because she'd been getting these headaches, the doctors wanted to be thorough and give her an MRI. We weren't really expecting anything to come of it; it just felt like a precaution. She had the scan on 23 December.

That Christmas, as usual, everyone had flown in for the holidays. We all went down to La Quinta and were preparing for a right old good time. I'd been sober for five years by this point; as soon as Tans got really sick the drink was over for me and we'd never been better.

On Christmas Eve, the phone call came. We took it together, away from the family. The news was terrible – there was cancer in her brain, now. The doctors were saying that in some ways it was more treatable than the ribs and the lungs, but it was hard to believe at that moment. In the next room, the family were all hanging out, chatting about this, that and the other, while we hid behind the bedroom door, crying in each other's arms.

Now we had to pull ourselves together, for the family. Tans was desperate that nothing would ruin the holiday she'd planned for everyone. We dried our eyes, kissed each other and walked out into the living room as though nothing had happened.

We didn't tell anyone that Christmas and New Year's what was going on. Tans, for her part, gave an amazing speech at Christmas lunch in which she urged everyone to enjoy every minute because we were so blessed to be together. She was crying happy tears, she said, because she was just so glad that everyone she loved was there.

I could hardly see straight for the agony of it.

Back in L.A., at Greenleaf Street in the New Year, Kaley was in Tans' walk-in closet while Tans was trying to find something to wear to go out. She told Kaley in a fairly off-handed way that they had found a little bit of cancer in her brain, but that they felt really confident that they could get it. Tans was once again very upbeat, but Kaley was smart enough that the words brain and cancer scared her. This felt different. Kaley knew that there were certain cancers – like pancreas, or brain – that frightened everyone the most because people didn't tend to beat them.

But Tans did everything to calm Kaley, saying that her radiation doctor was confident in the treatment, that the lung was actually less receptive to the treatment than the brain – all that kind of thing. There were apparently two baby lesions, and one bigger one, but the doctor thought he could get them . . .

Tans' bravery was sorely tested by her first radiation treatment on the brain. When she came out she was crying because it had been a very intensive thing. They had put a very tight cap on her skull and then they turned on the radiation – Tans said she could hear it zapping her in that very small room. She hated that treatment. It would take about eight minutes each time, four days a week, for about two weeks, then they would give her a break because they would want to see if it had done anything.

Then, like with the angiograms all those years, we'd have to wait to see what the outcome was. In the meantime, Tans would have to take a high dosage of steroids to protect the brain and to prevent seizures. But when the steroid dosage was lowered, in February 2019, seizures did start happening. One of the tumours was on part of the brain that controlled the left side of Tans' body, so when the seizures hit, she'd lose control of her left arm and hand and her speech was affected too. Tans would do her best to communicate with us with her eyes. We would take her yet again to Cedars-Sinai where the steroids would be increased and then Tans was allowed home, and the cycle continued. But all this would interfere with her chemo . . .

What you learn is that medical science is all about balancing risks and probabilities. Tans' doctors were wonderful in trying everything to make her comfortable, and we recognized how difficult their job was. Lower the steroids and the seizures hit; add the steroids back in and the side effects were horrible. Try to do some chemo but have to miss a treatment because of the seizures . . . truly, I don't know how Tans remained so positive and lovely.

Another of the side effects of all this was horrific leg pain, making sleep so difficult for her. Once again, she had to take fentanyl, which she described as 'a very dark drug'. And her treatment once again lowered her already low immune system and we'd have to take her back to the hospital with regular infections.

It just seemed so unfair that after everything, she was having to face all this. How much should one beautiful person have to take?

Most of 2018 and the early part of 2019 was a blur of doctors' appointments, radiation, tests, waiting, infections, ICU visits, and on and on. Sometimes, even though she wanted to be home, we felt that Tans was safer when she was in the hospital. We'd call the doctor when we weren't sure what to do and there was a tiny bit of relief if they said to bring her in, even though it was so hard on Tans. Through it all, though, Tans defined 'trooper'. She did everything she could to stay positive and hopeful, even in the face of these terrible diagnoses. We kept on with her heart medication, we kept on trying to be upbeat, we kept on in love.

Tans never spent a night alone.

Valentine's Day 2019 came and went. I think I knew it was our last but, at the same time, I didn't want to believe that this was our final chapter. Tans really tried that day, but she couldn't take in the stuff that I'd got her. It was the first time where there really was no point buying a Cartier bangle for her – she would have never worn it. We were running out of time. I got her a massive bunch of flowers and it was as much as she could do to smile that day.

And I got her a blow-up heart balloon on a fucking stick.

In my mind, I kept pushing it away. I would walk down

a street and want to scream, but I had to keep it together for everyone. When the plane you're on starts bumping and swooping, the first thing you do is look at the cabin crew to see if they're panicking. I was the airline staff in our lives; Tans and Kaley and her family were the passengers. If she looked at me and I was panicking, Tans would be frightened. And I couldn't have her frightened.

But yeah, sometimes on the way to golf I'd pull over and just scream.

Tans always said that if you want a doctor to look after you, allow them to see that you're a human and always be really nice to them. She was forever forming connections with her doctors and nurses. Tans was so extraordinary that no one would ever forget her in any case, but she always made the extra effort to be lovely to the people looking after her; it was just her way.

Her main doctor, Dr Rosenfelt, had been having some health issues of his own and she always made a point of asking him how he was feeling, how his wife was doing, where they were planning to go on holiday. He was a busy man and a serious doctor but he just couldn't help himself, so he'd hang around a bit and talk to her.

But each chemo would cause a setback requiring a blood transfusion or fluids, or she'd get another infection – Tans was so weak. Having to drive her back and forth to Cedars-Sinai in all that traffic and heat was horrendous; I don't know how Kaley managed it, but she'd really stepped in at this point.

Kaley had taken 2019 off work. She had dearly wanted

to look after her mummy, and in the last six months of her life, Kaley was our strength. It was almost as if Kaley felt that she was there when this all started and would see it through to the very end. Her bond with her mum was a spiritual one, I think. Perhaps it was because of the heart transplant – it made Tans the person she was and was part of Kaley's story from the start, and made the two of them like one person. Watching it from the outside, sometimes it looked like an out-of-body relationship; more than mother and daughter, it was like they'd fused through that early trauma into one person from two.

Dr Rosenfelt was worried that Tans' quality of life was now becoming subpar and in May 2019 it was he who first mentioned that perhaps hospice might be an option. Tans was so out of it on the fentanyl that Kaley doesn't think it quite registered. Kaley called me – I had unavoidably been in the UK at the time – and I had to call the doctor myself to hear what he had to say. I told Kaley that we'd keep going with the chemo, that we'd get through this together, all of us. I don't think I wanted to admit to what I was hearing.

Tans always felt safer when her own mum was around, so we flew her out. Then we flew Lou out too. These were signs of the final things.

Still there was one last attempt at chemotherapy. Tans was scheduled to do the second round of it on a Monday, but on the Saturday night she was showing signs of having another seizure. Kaley gave her an extra steroid, but then rightly decided to take Tans to the emergency room. Lauren went straight to the hospital from work, and then she too decided to take a leave of absence.

Kaley fell asleep in the room with Tans but was shaken awake by Dr Rosenfelt. He took her outside and quietly told her he thought Tans had about a month left to live. The last chemo was cancelled and then, when we were all together, we were invited to go to Cedars-Sinai for a meeting.

17

DAYS, WEEKS, MAYBE MONTHS

There's a room in Cedars-Sinai I hope you never have to see. Every hospital has that room. It's usually off to the side of a ward with chairs along each wall, a window if you're lucky. Maybe someone has hung some standard hospital pictures – mountains, a lake, a peaceful waterfall. There's no sign that it's ever used for patients: no treatment table covered in paper, no receptacle labelled 'SHARPS', no monitors, no bank of plug outlets, no sink, no otoscopes hanging from a hook. Just a room, a place to meet.

It's the worst room in the world.

The first time I went to Cedars-Sinai with Tans – years ago when she was first sick with cancer – I remember walking past that room. Tans was there to have laser treatment for her melanoma and, as I passed the room, I noticed that there was a group of people in there. They looked like one family and they were all crying, distraught, their heads in their hands, which I noticed were shaking. That day, all those years ago, I paused as I passed, looking through the little slit of the window in the door, and I thought,

'I never want to be in that room.' I said a little prayer then to something, someone, I don't know what. But I knew I never wanted to be in that room.

In June 2019, me, Lou, Maureen, and Kaley, were invited into that room. Same room, same shitty pictures on the wall, only this time they were accompanied by little thank-you drawings and paintings for the nurses and the doctors sent in by children. Five-year-olds, three-year-olds, eight-year-olds – all had daubed bits of white paper with thick finger paint – it felt like we were in an infants' classroom. Innocence, the beginnings of life, hope and security, play and simplicity, were all stuck to the walls of that room . . .

. . . In which we sat, surrounded by counsellors and doctors, who were talking as though Tanya Jones had already gone. So instead of being in an infants' classroom, in fact we were in the opposite side of life: the dark, painful, horrifying end of God's waiting room.

We arrived at Cedars-Sinai that day in one life. We went into that room and, when they were done talking to us, we left that room and walked into a completely different, new, terrifying life. We'd gone in one door and come out the same door but it was a million miles from where we'd entered.

The whole meeting took about 20 minutes.

Fifty feet away, down the corridor and to the right, Tans lay in her hospital bed, talking to Lauren. She kept asking Lauren why the doctors kept taking Kaley away? 'Why are they talking to her? Why aren't they talking to me?' Tans asked.

As I left that meeting room, I realized I was completely numb, as though I'd been given a massive dose of anaesthetic. My limbs were cold, my legs were weak; had I just run a marathon? No. I had just stood up and walked into the opposite part of life.

As those counsellors had talked to us, I had heard myself say 'OK . . . OK', but it wasn't going in, not registering in any part of my brain. I think they mentioned hospice, but she wasn't doing that, I knew – she was coming home. Simple as. But all you know is you're in that room that you never wanted to be in, and you know when you come out . . . You can never bring yourself around to what they've just told you.

What exactly had we been told? It hit us like a sledge-hammer. I can hardly bring the words to the page.

Days.

Weeks.

Maybe months.

We who loved her so had had to leave that room with those four words coursing through each of our hearts like poison, and we had to walk the 50 feet to where she slept, oblivious to the sentence she'd just been handed by the hateful, evil, unfair universe.

It was the longest 50 feet I'd ever walked in my entire life; I know that. Longer, more draining than any football match; harder, more painful than any training session; more terrifying than any fucking dance routine at the Royal Variety Performance. In the room, the grief had been horrific – so horrific that I don't know how I got the words out – but I had just about said to everyone, 'I just don't want her to know. I don't want her being scared.' Because, at that stage, there was no point her being scared; what was the point of that?

And then we four had walked to join her in her room, where she now slept, her body gently rising and falling with life. Lauren looked at us, then looked away. The cold world hadn't reached Tans, yet; she was surrounded by us: Her father, Lou, her hero, the man who'd walked her to a field more than four decades earlier and had pointed out a pony there that was hers to ride. Her mother, Maureen, who'd said 'Who is he?' the day after the night Tans and I had fallen in love. Her daughter, Kaley, who had been born at the start of her mother's second life, at the beginning of her second heart, and who had been her everything, every day, forever. Lauren, who had dropped everything and been there for us every single day, every single moment we needed her, so that she too was now family.

And me. Vincent Jones. The 12-year-old boy who became the man who loved her with a passion that still cannot dim and was not dimmed even by the merest amount on that day they'd told us 'days, weeks, maybe months'. Tanya had saved me and had shown me the unconditional love I had so craved for all my life. I was there, with her family, with our family, and I watched her sleeping, knowing those four evil words – 'days, weeks, maybe months' – were poisoning all of us, but knowing, too that we loved her purely and completely, as she had always loved us, and that no poisonous words could ever change that.

We had lived under the threat of death for the entirety of our relationship because of her heart. We never knew how much time she'd get, and certainly in the early days she would say, 'I'm not having another transplant.' Her new heart had been a trooper, though; it was strong to the end.

Whenever Tanya was scared, she'd say the same thing: 'I'm going to be alright. Vince here will look after me. You'll look after me, won't you?'

And every time I had said, 'Yes, I'll look after you.' And I always did.

But suddenly, and though I always knew this day would come, it was one step too far. I could no longer fulfil the promise I made every day to look after Tanya Jones. After all those years, I couldn't do it; it was out of my power. I couldn't stop any clocks, and I couldn't look after her, now. I couldn't save her.

We'd been in intensive care a couple of times with Tans before, and sometimes we'd had to face that maybe she wouldn't be coming out. Then she'd beat it, and she'd try and get back to a normal life. But now it was real and unbeatable.

In that last year, most days we were at a doctor or in a hospital. But she never lost her determination. In fact, Tans would get cross if I told her I was staying home. 'Go, play golf!' she'd insist, and she'd send Lou with me – 'Go look after Dad,' she'd say. And as sick as Tans was, she'd be determined to cook me dinner; I don't know how or why. And in 27 years, she never cooked me anything out the freezer – imagine that. Even to the end, she'd prepare something fresh and then she'd sit on the sofa and her ribs would hurt so much that she would have to go upstairs and lie down.

I'd gather her up and carry her upstairs as gently as I could, then once she was settled in bed I'd come down to clean up. But I could hear her upstairs watching TV. I'd be downstairs and this little girl upstairs ... I could hear her laughing at the TV show *Friends*, or old comedies like *Airplane* or *Naked Gun 2½*, even though she'd seem them umpteen times. She'd laugh and she was in so much pain.

In that room they'd told us her laughter would be ending, in days, weeks, or months.

One of the hardest things about that meeting in that room is that you talk for yourself, but you've got a daughter there, a mother there, a father there, a brother. I'm talking as the husband and I'm saying, 'Oh, I don't want her to know,' and I had to hope I was doing the right thing for everyone.

There were other decisions to make, too – terrible, awful, horrible decisions. Lou, understandably, had initially said, 'We're going to take her home.' He wanted to bury Tans with her Nanny Ella and her grandfather Tommy, whom Tans had idolized. I completely understood how he felt.

Then, Lou slept on it, and the next day he came to me and said, 'You know what, she needs to be here with you and Kaley.' I can't imagine the size of his heart, its depth, to be able to say that. Lou is a man's man; he'll probably die with quite a few bloke's secrets. You can tell him something and that's that and it's buried with Lou. That's who he is. But here he was, able to put aside his coming grief for the good of his granddaughter and son-in-law. Kaley was settled in the US and that's where she and Lauren were planning to be for the rest of their lives; I never know where my road's going to go, but ultimately, I'll probably end up here. So that's where Lou thought his daughter should be, too.

These are the decisions which that room in Cedars-Sinai, and in hospitals around the world, force you to make. Should someone know? Where should someone be laid to rest? How will we live without her? We sat around her bed, waiting for her to wake up, knowing what we now knew. There would be hundreds of decisions to come – could we take her home, could we give her the care she needed, could we make her comfortable, could we keep the fear from her, could we give her hope, even though our hope had been dashed by that room?

Tans would come home – that much we knew. We could nurse her, Kaley could nurse her, we'd make do.

Years earlier, Tans had needed regular morphine injections and she faced being hospitalized for them. To get her home, I had to be the one to inject her, otherwise they would have kept her in. Not in my wildest dreams did I think I could ever have put a needle in someone. But there I was, injecting her in the mornings and in the evenings, with the needle in her belly. We did it so long that her whole midsection was just little dots.

I had become someone who had to inject his wife with morphine. I never batted an eyelid in the end. I would have done anything to take away her pain, to make her safe.

'I'm going to be alright. Vince here will look after me.

You'll look after me, won't you?' That was what she always said. And it had been true, right up until that day in that room in Cedars-Sinai. The room I never wanted to see.

Later that evening, Tans stirred, then she woke, and then, as ever, she rallied, and I have her on video going across the room behind her walker, saying, 'I'm going home. I'm going home.'

There are some things you cannot look at straight on. Imagine a fire, or a star exploding, or the sun suddenly appearing right outside your window. This is what we all saw that night: Tanya Jones walking to and fro in a cramped hospital room, chanting that she was going home. The burning heat of the moment makes me want to scream still.

Only one tiny moment of joy came from that meeting in that room in Cedars-Sinai. While we'd been discussing Tans' care, Lauren had taken the opportunity to ask Tans if she could marry Kaley. Even in the darkest moments, there can be light. You just have to fill the holes with love.

18

THE EARTHQUAKE

One of the hardest things about Tans being on hospice at home was that the care she was given by visiting doctors and nurses naturally didn't involve anything to do with prolonging life. But we still kept on with her heart medication; it would have felt wrong to not do so. We'd been all about it for our entire relationship – every morning, every evening. We weren't about to stop now.

All Tans wanted to do was plan Christmas 2019. I think she wanted another milestone to get to – as long as she felt she could get there, she would have crawled on her hands and knees to do it. 'Right, I want to book my mum and dad's flights now,' she'd say. 'I want Shane and Amy,' (her niece). 'Right. Let's get Belle sorted out. Let's get the flights.' Belle is Steve Terry's daughter from his new relationship, but she is part of our family – she called Tans 'Mummy'. 'I want us to celebrate New Year's Eve. I don't want to celebrate our anniversary now,' she said. 'I want to do it on New Year's Eve, when we're all together. We can celebrate our anniversary when I'm not in the hospital.' She was forever looking forward.

Tans also never lost her sense of humour, either. Around that time, she whispered to me, 'You've got to promise me, Vincent, that if anything ever happens and they come to get me, make sure I've got my underwear on.'

I'm proud to say that my son, Aaron, and I are best mates. He's got two children, making me a grandad twice over – six and two, they are now. He's served in the military and now he's training to be a pilot in Ireland; I couldn't be prouder of him.

But disaster has struck his family, too. In the middle of June 2019, I was in Ireland burying my new granddaughter, who had died at birth. To see your son and his wife put a tiny white box in the ground . . . I've never seen grief like it. There's something so wrong, so upside down about a parent having to bury a child; it's the world in reverse, it's against natural law.

It's the hardest thing there is.

By late June, when the doctors came in to see her at home, Tans was very weak. But she'd still find the energy to say, 'I'm married to this beautiful boy. He's very complex, but he's very beautiful, and he's my boyfriend.' Our wedding anniversary was 25 June. Leading up to it, if anyone came in – nurses, doctors, anyone – Tans would say, 'It's my wedding anniversary in a few days. I've been married to my boyfriend for 25 years.' And, as ever, even at her most poorly, when I left the room, I'd throw her that kiss and she'd catch it.

Despite the terrible times, we also tried to look forward. Kaley and Lauren needed their own place and Tans was so excited about the prospect of them finding a house. Tans had been looking at real estate during the early months of 2019; she wanted to find us a plot of land to build on where we could settle and she wanted Kaley and Lauren to find their first home together too. In fact, she would sit for hours looking at houses for Kaley, every evening. She'd show the brochures she been given to everybody in the UK on Face-Time. Some nights, I'd wake up and find her awake next to me, and she'd ask to see the real estate listings again, which she kept by the bed.

Lauren and Kaley would sit at the foot of her bed and talk with her about houses for hours. She would reminisce about all the houses she'd lived in – Gaddesden Crescent, Hunter's Oak, Redbourn, Box Lane, Cedars in Tring, Shootersway, Mulholland – and tell stories. For her, this was one of the most special things: making a home. And yet I knew she'd meant it when she said she'd live in a caravan as long as we were together. In May, Tans seemed even just about well enough to actually look at one of the houses that Kaley and Lauren were thinking of buying, but it was a struggle to get her there and, after that, we just knew that it was too much for her.

One day, about a week before the end, and with everyone around her in the bed – Lou, Maureen, Lauren, Kaley – Tans looked at me and said, 'We've been married 25 years and we've been together 27 years. Isn't that amazing? I'm still crazy mad in love, giddy mad in love, and that's rare after 27 years.'

Lou stroked her face. The world span at a different speed

than usual. There was too much air in the room, and not enough. This woman who had saved so many people . . . I'd promised her I'd look after her and not let anything bad happen to her, and here we were, watching as the cruel world let its grip on her loosen.

Tans was still thinking she could beat it, even then. The doctors had always said that she was the strongest person they've ever met.

I got a call a few years ago from Angie, a sister of my lifelong friend, Seamus. Seamus had been in Harefield awaiting a new heart. In the call, Angie said, 'Vin, I don't know if you ever knew this, but I went in to see Seamus a couple of years ago. Tanya was sitting on the bed holding his hand talking to him.' Tans had never told me. That's who she was; that's the perfect Tanya Jones story.

Now we were sitting on the bed holding her hand. I couldn't leave her side. Tans often said, 'Vin's got a good heart. You've got to trust him. He has got a good heart.'

I had given her so many reasons to not think that and yet she never wavered. She saw the 12-year-old boy and she loved him unconditionally, right up to this moment, when he couldn't save her as he'd promised he would. It was one more way I'd let her down, but even I couldn't change this, though I still held out a glimmer of hope. That's what humans do; that's what love does. You never give in – you can't. Your body and your mind won't let you.

I flew Tans' best friends, Julie and Joanne, over to see her. They'd both lost dear people in their lives and they knew what was what. I was still talking about how we were going

216

to get Tans over this and how she was going to recover, but Julie and Joanne could see something different. They said, 'She's not going to make it through the weekend, Vin.' That was the cold light of day, right there.

I flew Shane over, too – the man who'd played his guitar in pubs and restaurants and at parties and who never looked up from his strumming without seeing his sister singing along to every fucking word – his biggest fan. By now, Tans was sleeping a lot, but when he arrived, she woke up and she was chatting nonstop for half an hour. Tans was so happy to see him.

At the end of every night, for as long as she was able, Tans would walk to the landing of the house and yell for everyone – mum, dad, Shane. They would come out of their rooms and meet her on the landing and she'd say, 'I just want to say goodnight.' That's what they used to do when she and Shane were little – the two kids would sit on the landing and sing songs together, and then mum and dad would come out and say goodnight and everyone would go off to bed.

Kaley had taken 2019 off of work to be with her mum full time. By the end, she would feed her mum a couple of spoons of rice pudding and sprinkle some of her meds on it; or she'd just sit holding her hand.

The week before Tans died, the hospice people said, 'It's not worth her taking her heart medication anymore.'

That was crushing. Those medications had always been within arm's reach, for 27 years. Now, they were of no use.

And then June turned into July. On Thursday 4 July,

Independence Day, we were all up in Tans' room when a massive earthquake hit – the Ridgecrest earthquake was the biggest in living memory for most of us. It originated about 120 miles north of L.A. and measured as much as 7.1 on the Richter scale (that's a lot). It was crazy in that room, there, with Tans, as her life ebbed and the whole house rocked.

Strong aftershocks from the earthquake hit again on Friday 5 July. Even the very earth couldn't let her go.

I was holding her when she was taking her last breaths.

I felt the pain leave her. It had been six years of pain, but now it was flying away, Tinker Bells of pain flying from her body.

I felt Tanya leave.

Tanya Jones died on Saturday 6 July 2019, surrounded by everyone she loved and everyone who loved her. She was 53 years old, and she was 32 years old.

And she was everything.

19

THE WHITE LIGHT

The night Tans died we were all sitting outside in the back garden at Greenleaf – it was around midnight, a still, overcast night, no moonlight. One by one, people were heading inside to bed, and I told them I'd be in in a little while. I wanted to smoke and watch the darkness and be alone.

On the wind, I could smell the night-blooming jasmine, a scent everyone associates with Los Angeles. There's really nothing like it; sweet and strong and beautiful; I always knew I was home when I smelled it.

That night, the scent was everywhere, and it mixed with my smoke until I was going mad with grief. These were the first moments of a new life, and I didn't want them; I didn't want any of it.

As I sat there, I noticed above me a white light. I knew it couldn't be a star because of the cloud cover, but there it was – a simple white light above me. I already knew that when you lose someone you can start to look for things, for signs, so I was on guard. I never believed in any of that stuff and I wasn't about to start now, even though my grief was stronger than the earth below me.

But that white light was there, and there was no denying it. It definitely wasn't a star and it wasn't a helicopter, or a plane, it was too low. I've since checked and re-checked the weather forecast for that night and it was overcast in Los Angeles on the night of 6 July; the sun didn't appear until noon the next day.

To the darkness I said, 'Well, that's a bit bizarre.' And I don't know why – as I said, I really don't believe in this stuff – but in my grief and desperation I said to the light, 'Is that you, babe?'

The light shone above me; it didn't waver, or change. Was it Tans? There was only one way to find out. I thought about all the times she'd say, 'Where's my kiss?' and I'd throw her one to catch. So that's what I did, right there in that dark garden – I threw one last kiss up to the white light above me, the light that wasn't a star or the moon or a plane or anything I recognized.

Suddenly, the light swerved, and dipped, and hovered, and then it flew – zoom! – it flew and swerved and then it disappeared away from me in that garden, with the jasmine blooming all around me, and left me, once again alone.

One of my first phone calls after Tanya died was to Dennis Byatt. He was the poor man whose wife and child had died years ago, and whose absence had allowed me to briefly play for Wealdstone, which had led to so many opportunities for me in my life.

Dennis said, 'I've been waiting for this call.'

'What do I do now, Den?' I said.

Dennis paused, and then he said, 'The only thing you can do, mate, the only thing I'll tell you to do, is make your own decisions. There will be people telling you to do this, to do that, this is right, that's wrong, why have you done this, and why have you done that. And if you go with what everybody else wants, you'll be disappointed later on. You just have to make your own decisions; go with how you feel.'

So that's what I did. I let Kaley organize the funeral; I felt it was hers to do, given the extraordinary bond she shared with Tans. And Kaley put together a beautiful service.

We had figured there might be 30 or 40 or so people at the service, but how wrong we were. I had stopped a few from flying over – it was too much to ask. But folks came anyway. Wally Downes, my mate from Wimbledon, flew in, attended the funeral and flew out the same day – can you imagine? Tans had always stuck up for him and they would text each other back and forth with silly videos he found to make her laugh. Jason Statham and Rosie Huntington-Whiteley came. Everyone from my golf club came, too. In the end there must have been at least 300 people there; it was standing room only. Tans had touched so many lives.

I looked at Maureen and Lou that day, and it just felt so unfair. As with Aaron and his wife having to bury their baby, it's just wrong when parents lose their child. It's out of nature.

Whenever Shane played a show, he would always sing 'Everything I Own' by Bread. A lot of people probably think that's a romantic love song, but it's actually about the song-writer, David Gates, missing his late father and wanting him back alive. Tans would sob when Shane sang it. But now it was all topsy-turvy – Lou had lost his daughter and I know he would have given everything he owned for another day with Tans. We all would have.

Kaley and Shane organized three slide shows, detailing the key parts of Tans' life, backed by the songs we loved – one was of me and Tans, one of Kaley and Tans and the other was of Tans with all her friends and family. People were heaving with sobs, as you can imagine. Kaley was also able to stand up and read a note she'd gotten from her mum – it basically said that she hoped Kaley was lucky enough to have found what she found: unlimited true love.

Kaley was so strong that day. She had picked up her mother's legacy, wrapped it around her and that's what's kept her going. But still I had to ask her how she had managed it.

Kaley said, 'It was Mummy speaking through me.'

About three months after Tansy left us, I went on *Good Morning Britain* to talk about her and what we'd been through. I did it because I wanted to show people that it's OK to grieve, it's OK to talk about loss and it's important to share stories of your loved ones when they go. I don't know how I got through it, to be honest, but then, I wasn't ashamed to cry. I felt like Tans was there with me and I hoped that by just being honest I'd reach some other people who'd gone through a loss. And I hoped she'd be proud of me, too. This was her legacy coming out through me.

Tans was forever helping someone, that was just her way, so for me to be able to go on that show and hear afterwards that I'd helped a few people – well, that made it all worth it. I did hear from a lot of people, actually, and I hope they all know that I get it, I truly do, and will always get it. I wish I didn't, but I know that Tans would insist on me looking outside of my grief to connect with people who need support; that's what she always did, and that's what I'm trying to do.

A little while after, I went on *Celebrity X Factor*, which of course gave everyone the chance to have a free hit at me. How could he do that, having just lost his wife, they asked? Well, Tans had been eager for me to do it – she loved it when I performed like that and urged me on to be a part of that show.

So I was determined I was going to make Tans proud, but more than that, this is why I did it: when I was on the stage, even if it was filled with dancers and musicians, I was actually alone up there, and there was only one person sitting in the audience. All the other seats were empty, but Tans was sitting there, right in the middle, and she was waiting for me backstage too.

X Factor kept me busy – it drove me on. Kaley would call twice, three times a week, and say, 'Just be you, be cool. Don't let yourself down.' And that's what I did. It was all to give Tans a smile and to make Kaley proud, like all those years ago on *Top of the Pops*.

It wasn't for Simon Cowell. I was grateful to him that he let me join at the last minute, but no, it wasn't for the judges. That was for Kaley, and my Tanya.

20

JOYOUS GRIEF

We are Tans now. She remains in the differences she's made to our lives. Every time we choose something better, kinder, more caring, that's her. That's what eternity means. Her physical form has gone, and we miss her constantly. The smile, the laughter, her voice, the way she looked back over her shoulder at us, the constant caring and nurturing and listening. All those things are gone, yes, but she saved us and so every time we're better people, we're emitting a dose of her into the world. But that doesn't mean it's not crushingly sad, every minute of every day.

After she went, so many little moments brought me to my knees. We cleaned out the house on Greenleaf – we couldn't stay a second in that place after we lost Tans, so we moved to a different house 15 minutes east – and I said to Kaley, 'This is the first time in 27 years her medicine hasn't been in the bathroom or by the bed.' It's all I'd ever known.

How to turn that grief into a joyous grief? That's the test now – how to turn this huge negative into something positive. I don't have all the answers, but I have a few.

First, tears. There have been so many tears, some public, lots private. There's nothing wrong with that; I have no shame in crying about Tans. She wouldn't want me to be crying all the time, but when it hits, I just let it out.

Then, I keep contact with her. I speak to her a lot. I still have a chat with her all the time – and you have to do that. You have to carry that with you.

I try to be kind and supportive of the people I love. Also, I'm not afraid to laugh and joke, however hard it is. Tans would have insisted; she was the life and soul of every gathering. That's what she'd want – even when my head is saying it's wrong.

As time goes on, each week, each month, different memories have come back to me, which is wonderful. That's helping build the joyous grief. You can't just curl up in a ball and let the world trample all over you. That would have devastated Tans. Our job now is to look after each other as best we can. That was Tans' wish.

But the central point of joyous grief for me is that Tans gave us all a task to do after she was gone, and we're trying to do it each day. We each have someone we have to care for, to look after, to love, someone whose dreams we have to try and bring to life. We have to find the positive in life and we have to move forward – always move forward. I'm going to make sure Kaley is settled, and Lauren is going to look after her, too. Kaley looks after me; I make sure Lou and Maureen are OK. Kaley calls them all the time, they call her.

Shane sent me a copy of the videos he and Kaley made

for the funeral, and I let myself have a cry. I was on my own, I had my little cry, but it was a joyous cry. Grief can be joyous as well as heartbreaking. When you're watching videos and you're looking at the pictures, you can just let your memories flood in – the good memories. I had 27 years with Tans so for me the final equation is a completely positive one – she was fantastic and our relationship was fantastic. This doesn't mean I don't cry; but I'm starting to cry happier tears.

We get all this from Tans; she was the one who set the tone for life after she left us. She is the core of joyous grief: we make decisions based on what she would have wanted, what she would have asked of us, what she would have insisted we care about. Tans wasn't a taskmaster – she was just a very loving, caring person, and she made people better around her. This gives us joy, to have been in the presence of that for so long. Our job now is to make sure we choose the right thoughts, ones that will ensure we do the right thing for each other. We're Tans' proxy, now; she can't be here anymore, but that doesn't mean we can't keep her alive by being there for each other, like she was always there for us. That's joyous grief; that's what we're up to now.

Kaley said it best: her mum was the definition of joyous, no matter what she was going through, so we have to honour that as a value in our lives, something we make a part of what we stand for as people. Tanya Jones was joyous, despite going through the most horrific things one can endure as a human. So, we have to find strength like she did to live with the same light and joy that she had. We have to live like she is watching and listening, and we have to have blind faith in that, or else we would fall apart.

She wrote out a poem for Kaley that said don't spend your years shedding wild tears but reach your hand out to others in cheer. And that was Kaley's mum: always reaching her hand out in cheer to each of us, to everyone, in fact, no matter how much pain she was experiencing, no matter what we'd put her through, no matter how lousy she felt. Tans focused on us at every turn and it alleviated *her* pain and *her* tears. This is our survival guide now – this is the survival guide she created for us to move forward in joy. We can learn how to cope by remembering how she did it; that's the great lesson, the great gift she left us.

And that's what I urge others to find in their lives. Yes, we've lost someone so, so special, but we are her now; we can embody who she was. We can learn from her, even though she's physically gone. What a gift she was. That gives me so much joy, even as I pull the car over and cry for the missing of her.

And I focus on what me and Tans were – that's a great comfort. Someone said to me, 'What made you two so strong?' And I said, 'I think we were two swans. Swans partner for life and I think we were swans.' I'm content with that. I'm very content with that.

I know she's gone, physically, but at the same time, I feel a glow around me. Sometimes I think, 'Come on, is that you?' It gives me comfort. A tiny bit of joy.

Others feel it, too. It was Maureen's birthday recently,

and a while back Tans had bought them a tea at the Grove Hotel in Hertfordshire but hadn't been well enough to do it. Maureen finally went to redeem the tea this year and, as she was leaving, there was the golf cart that used to drive us all around when it rained. Maureen just texted, 'That bloody golf cart!' I was able to write back, 'You know somebody who would have a great big smile on her face today.' These are the little moments we cherish, the tiny messages from the universe that perhaps we're not completely alone.

Sometimes I find myself being a little angry at what I call the wasted years of the drinking, when I let myself down and upset her so badly. But all the time I knew a better person was in there, and Tans knew it too. That's an incredible thing to take with me, every day. That someone believed in me. It makes everything fall into a perspective I can live with.

My advice to anyone going through this is to keep busy and go and talk to someone.

I'm so tired, though – I'm so tired that I can't get excited about anything. That's not like me. I can't get a buzz. If I just checked my numbers now and had won the Euro millions, I don't think you'd see a different expression on my face. If a truck came towards me in the street, I'm not sure I'd be able to dive out of the way. They say depression is anger without energy; well, I guess I have that.

I'm really, really irritable, too. I'm very quick and short tempered. It feels like . . . like confusion. I don't know.

All I can say is if you've got problems and you think

that the weight is too heavy, you have to go and speak to somebody.

And if you need to leave, like we did from our house, Greenleaf, then just leave the place.

I know Tans' love will get me through this. I'm looking after Kaley for her, but I'm not ready to do much else – I'm not at that stage yet. I still want to hide a little bit. I think, 'Just leave me with her for a minute. Let us have our moment. I'm not done with our moment.'

And I don't know how long it will take for that feeling to change. That's a very private thing. Sure, I've got to run around being busy, doing X Factor, and acting, and the tours, and playing golf, and everything. But that's my brave face, an art face that I put on, every time I leave the house. I have an entertainer's suit and a grief suit. I take the art face and the entertainer's suit off at night and I sadly don the others, when I'm alone and Tans isn't there.

What's happened to our family is too big to really get our heads around. Recently I said to Kaley, 'Right. You know, I feel we're moving on a little bit now,' and as I said it, I thought, 'Of course we're not.'

Of course we're not. There's no moving on.

I'm going to get through this, though – that's the thing. But grief is not like a sweet wrapper in the wind – it's not going to flit off and go further and further away. And it's not like a boat going under the bridge downstream – it's not going to go away out of sight. So that's why I say I'm trying to build a joyous grief and really embrace the great love that Tans and I had, and build on it and strive off it, and that's where my energy will come from.

And we need to fulfil Tans' wishes. If we can keep moving forward – a house, maybe a baby one day for Lauren and Kaley, god willing – then her final wishes will come true, and that's not nothing.

I saw that little girl's face today when we were walking around that house. That, there, is everything now. That's her mother, shining through Kaley, smiling at me, a little girl aged 11 or 12 in Sun Sports in Watford, a lifetime ago, before all this happened, before before before.

Epilogue:
THE HOUSE IN VAN NUYS

It sits in the north-west corner of a quiet cul-de-sac in Van Nuys, a neighbourhood about half an hour from where we live now. There's a little yard out front, leading to the garage; the house itself sits back a bit at the end of a sloping driveway. Inside there are three bedrooms, two bathrooms. It's about twelve hundred square feet. There's a big kitchen with plenty of space for Lauren, who's a professional chef, to create her magic. At the back there's a closed-in porch which looks out over a big yard, which boasts a cabana kind of thing, with a built-in grill and barstools and a TV.

This was the one last thing we had to complete, one last promise we'd made to Tans. We'd spent months looking and making offers and getting out-bid, but still we tried. And then we found the house in Van Nuys, Kaley made the offer and – boom.

We used the money we made when we sold Hunter's Oak, the place where it all really began for the three of us. And maybe when Kaley moves in, it will lighten the grief a bit more, because it's something else that we've fulfilled for her. Maybe I'll be able to look up into the sky and imagine Tans' smile, the one I lived with for 27 years.

Now it's up to me to let go a bit and let Kaley and Lauren fly.

I've done up a lot of houses and I love it, but I have to let them do it their way. I went to the new house with them and in my head I made a list. I want to change the doors, paint this, paint that, knock that wall out, knock this wall out – but it has to come from them. I have to stand back; it's got to be all their own decisions.

As I write, Kaley and Lauren have just left to go to Home Depot to look at light fixtures and bedroom stuff and bathroom stuff. It's what me and Tans always did. It's déjà vu.

I'm alone in this rental, near my golf club, in Los Angeles, in early 2020. It's been a good, beautiful day in California. I played golf with my dear friends, made some silly Instagram movies and larked about, though I shot a much higher score than I used to – I just don't have the drive, literally and figuratively, right now. It'll come back I suppose; who knows? And maybe I'll stay in Los Angeles; maybe I'll move back to the UK full time. I'll land wherever I land. I always have. Until one day I land back with Tanya, wherever she is in the universe.

Will I be happy in three years, or six years, nine? Who knows? All I know is I am getting nearer to those pearly gates. I'm going to entertain Tans for a little while until I get there.

Tansy has been gone seven months today.

We're busy getting work done on Kaley and Lauren's house, and we aim to have it finished by 14 April, Tans' birthday. Kaley and Lauren will sleep in the house for the first time that night, and wake up on Kaley's birthday, 15 April.

I've got to look after this beautiful spirit that Tans brought into this world. I've got to see it through, now, until this little girl is in her new house with her partner. Then, hopefully, in the near future, there will be three of them living there (plus their little dog), and I'll be over there cooing and singing 'Where Do You Go to My Lovely' to my grandchild – no, to *our* grandchild – and telling that little boy or girl all about their grandmother, Tanya Jones, my Tans, and how she was the most wonderful person who ever lived.

Acknowledgements

Myself and my daughter Kaley, who helped me write this book, would like to thank the following: Lou Lamont, Maureen Lamont, Shane Lamont, Lauren Keefe, Julie McGregor, Joanne Southern, Harefield Hospital, Dr Andrew Mitchell, Sir Magdi Yacoub, Cedars-Sinai Hospital, Dr Fred Rosenfelt, Luke Dempsey, Vicky Eribo, Alex Segal at Inter-Talent Rights Group and Alex Cole at Elevate Entertainment.

Vinnie Jones is a British actor and former professional footballer who played as a midfielder from 1984 to 1999, most notably for Wimbledon, Leeds United, Sheffield United, Chelsea, QPR and Wales. Vinnie Jones and his wife Tanya were together for twenty-seven years, married for twenty-five. In July 2019, Tanya lost her fight with cancer and passed away at home, surrounded by her family.

Vinnie has written this book with the help and support of his daughter, Kaley, as a tribute to Tanya. Vinnie is also the author of *Vinnie Jones: The Autobiography* and *It's Been Emotional*.